STRETCHING EXERCISES FOR SENIORS OVER 60

Unleash Your Vitality, Stay Active, and Embrace Life: Essential Stretching Exercises Tailored for Vibrant Seniors Over 60

Michael Stratch

© Copyright 2023. All rights reserved.

No portion of the 'Stretching Exercises for Seniors over 60' may be replicated or disseminated in any form without the written consent of the copyright owner, Michael Stratch, except for certain uses permitted under copyright law.

Table of Contents

INTRODUCTION 7

CHAPTER 1: **UNDERSTANDING THE AGING BODY** 9

   AGING AND THE MUSCLES, BONES, AND JOINTS 9
      Aging and Your Bones 9
      Aging and Your Joints 10
      Aging and Your Muscles 11
   BENEFITS OF STRETCHING 13

CHAPTER 2: **GETTING STARTED SAFELY** 15

   WHAT TO KNOW ABOUT EXERCISING AS A SENIOR 15
   WARMING UP 18
      Shoulder Rolls 19
      Neck Stretches 21
      Lateral Arm Swings 22
      Wrist Circles 23
      Leg Swings 24
      Lateral Leg Swings 25
      Ankle Circles from a Sitting Position 26
      Seated Hamstring Stretch 27
      Knee Bends 28
   THE BENEFITS OF WARMING UP 29
   HOW LONG AND OFTEN SHOULD YOU WARM UP? 30

CHAPTER 3: **ESSENTIAL STRETCHING EXERCISES** 31

   NECK 31
      Neck Flexion 32
      Neck Flexion Assisted 33
      Neck Extension 34

  Neck Extension Assisted 35

  Neck Lateral Flexion 36

  Neck Rotation 37

  Cervical Stars 38

 Back 40

  Door-Assisted Side Bend 40

  Wall-Assisted Upper-Back Stretch 42

  Head-Tilted Forward Bend 43

  Bear Hug 44

 Shoulders & Chest 45

  Posterior Arm Cradle 45

  Arm Circles 47

  Wall-Assisted Chest Opener 48

  Bent-Arm Fly 50

  Elbow Circles 52

  Extended Palm Press 53

  Crisscross Arms 54

  Shoulder Circles 55

 Arms, Wrists, & Hands 57

  Wall-Assisted Bicep Stretch 57

  Tricep Stretch 59

  Wrist Flexion 61

  Wall-Assisted Forearm Stretch 62

  Prayer Hands 63

  Finger Stretch 65

  Thumb Stretch 67

 Core & Hips 69

  Hip Twist 69

  Triangle Pose 71

  Seated Spinal Twist 72

  Side Lunge 73

Legs, Knees, Feet & Ankles 75
- *Toe Touch Standing* 75
- *Standing Quadricep Stretch* 77
- *Foot Sickle* 78
- *Toe Stretch* 79
- *High Knee Walking* 80
- *Ankle Circles* 81
- *Wall-Assisted Calf Stretch* 83
- *Forward Lunge* 85

CHAPTER 4: BUILDING BALANCE AND STABILITY 87

The Advantages of Balance Training 87
Balance Exercises 89
- *Side Leg Raise* 89
- *Forward Heel Taps* 90
- *Side Toe Taps* 91
- *Heel Raise* 93
- *Toe Raise* 94
- *Lean Forward* 95
- *Seated Arm Lifts* 96
- *Seated Arm and Leg Lifts* 97
- *Torso Rotation Leg Openers* 98
- *Forward Reach to the Ankle Tap* 100

CHAPTER 5: STRENGTHENING FOR A RESILIENT BODY 101

Benefits of Strength Training 101
Strength Exercises 102
- *Forward Lunge* 102
- *Lateral Lunge* 103
- *Bent-Over Row* 105
- *Reverse Fly* 107
- *Shoulder Press* 109

Iron Cross *111*

Upright Row *113*

CHAPTER 6: CUSTOMIZING YOUR ROUTINE 115

DEVELOPING A PERSONALIZED STRETCHING ROUTINE 115

SAMPLE ROUTINE 117

TRACKING PROGRESS 119

REWARDING YOURSELF 120

CONCLUSION 121

APPENDIX 122

ADDITIONAL RESOURCES 122

GLOSSARY OF TERMS 123

FREQUENTLY ASKED QUESTIONS 124

Introduction

Welcome to " Stretching Exercises for Seniors over 60"! It is with great pleasure and admiration that I warmly greet you, fellow adventurers on the path of healthy living in the golden years. Your dedication to maintaining an active lifestyle is truly commendable, and it is my sincere belief that the journey we embark on together through this book will be both enriching and empowering.

Like many of you, I have experienced the joys and challenges that come with aging gracefully. Throughout my life, I have been passionate about health and wellness, and I am incredibly humbled to be sharing my knowledge and experiences with you.

As we navigate the pages of this book, I want you to know that my journey is not that of a distant expert, but rather that of a companion on the same path. I, too, have faced the inevitable changes that come with age, and it is through these experiences that I've come to understand the immense value of flexibility for seniors over 60.

Flexibility is not just a physical attribute; it is the key that unlocks the door to a vibrant and fulfilling life. Through stretching exercises tailored for your needs, you can enhance your overall well-being, maintain independence, and savor the richness of life at every stage.

At the heart of this book lies the recognition that our bodies may slow down with age, but our spirits need not follow suit. In fact, it is during these later years that we have the opportunity to embrace new passions, cultivate lasting friendships, and rediscover the essence of who we are. By adopting a regular stretching routine, you open the door to a world of possibilities, where limitations become stepping stones to growth.

In this book, we will explore various stretching routines that cater specifically to seniors, taking into account the unique challenges and triumphs that accompany this phase of life.

Stretching not only improves flexibility but also plays a crucial role in enhancing overall mobility and balance. As we age, the risk of falls increases, and the fear of losing independence looms large. However, by incorporating regular stretches into your daily routine, you build a sturdy foundation that bolsters your stability and reduces the likelihood of accidents.

Beyond the physical benefits, stretching also serves as a gateway to mental clarity and emotional well-being. Engaging in mindful stretches fosters a sense of inner peace, allowing you to embrace the present moment and let go of unnecessary worries. Moreover, as you connect with your body and movements, you'll find yourself better equipped to handle stress and navigate life's challenges with grace and resilience.

As we progress through this journey together, I encourage you to approach each stretch with a curious and open heart. The path may not always be smooth, but remember that every effort you invest in your well-being is an investment in a life well-lived. Celebrate the small victories, for they are stepping stones towards greater accomplishments.

Let this book be your guide on this path to vitality and fulfillment. Together, we will celebrate the freedom of movement, cherish the joy of progress, and revel in the triumphs of staying active as we gracefully embrace the journey of life.

Chapter 1:
Understanding the Aging Body

As you age, your body undergoes certain processes that you have no direct control over. These biological events are a natural part of the aging process in human beings. In this chapter, we will focus on enlightening you about what happens in your body as you age. This knowledge is crucial because it enhances your understanding regarding why training should be a crucial part of your everyday lifestyle. The information that you will get in this chapter will give you reasons that serve as a footing for engaging in an active lifestyle.

Aging and the Muscles, Bones, and Joints

As human beings age, there are changes that happen to their posture and walking patterns. Usually, these changes are attributed to alterations that take place in the bones, joints, and muscles as years go by.

Aging and Your Bones

The skeleton that supports your body is made up of bones that are connected together through joints. When you are young, your bones are strong and so is the skeleton. As a result, your body posture is straight and uncompromised. This state changes as your body tends to get weaker with age. You might find it progressively difficult to keep your spinal cord straight. In fact, you may experience immense pain in your back if you try to. In some cases, the bones don't only get weaker as you age, they might become brittle, and this can result in them potentially being easier to break. While bones can sometimes break as a result of injuries, brittle bones simply fracture without any reasonable cause. This, of course, significantly affects your walking patterns and posture.

The bones that make up your spinal cord are known as the vertebrae. These bones are arranged in such a way that there is a gel-like substance called hyaluronic acid located between each of them. The role of this substance is to cushion the vertebrae, as well as maintain the size of your trunk. The trunk is the region of your body that is located below your head and just before your legs. As age catches up with you, the gel-like cushion loses fluid, thereby making the vertebrae appear shorter.

The result of this change is a shorter trunk. The mineral content of the spine bones also reduces with age. All these changes contribute to a curved and compressed spinal cord, something which is quite common among the elderly.

Conditions Associated With the Bones

Now that you have an idea of some of the things that happen in your body as you age, let's have a quick rundown of the conditions that tend to emerge as you age. In this section, we will focus more on the conditions that affect your bones.

- **Osteoporosis:** It is normal for bone mass and density to reduce with a corresponding increase in age. This is especially true for women who are in their menopause. Science has it that bone density tends to remain stable for age ranges between 25 and 50 years (Johns Hopkins Medicine, 2022). Beyond 50 years of age, bone formation begins to take place at a pace that is slower than the rate at which they break down. This results in reduced mass and density of the bones in the long run.
- **Osteophytes:** Osteophytes happens when finger joints lose their cartilage, and the bones get slightly thicker.

Aging and Your Joints

Walking patterns are also affected by unhealthy joints. Your flexibility and ease of movement is a factor of good and able joints. The reason why your bones do not rub against each other as you walk is the presence of synovial membranes and fluids that surround the joints. These fluids lubricate the joint area to reduce any form of friction that might possibly occur. The amount of synovial fluid that is available in your joint areas may reduce as you grow older. This means that the probability of your bones brushing against each other as you move becomes elevated. Walking becomes more difficult and even painful. This is part of what takes away the joy of most senior citizens as they fail to move without external support.

Your joints are also cushioned by what is known as cartilage, which covers the ends of your bones. They are there to further protect your bones from rubbing against each other. The older you grow, the more these cartilages begin to wear away, thereby exposing the ends of your bones. This condition is called arthritis and it adds to the uncomfortable feelings that senior citizens might experience in their joints as they walk. Loss of cartilage is quite common on the hip and knee joints.

In joints around the shoulders, minerals may accumulate on the joints, a process that is known as calcification.

Aging and Your Muscles

Your muscles also play major roles in enhancing your movements. They provide the strength and force that you need for movement to happen. However, aging comes with reduced vigor as the muscles grow weaker, too. Medically, the condition in which muscle function is lost as a result of aging is called 'sarcopenia'. This word originates from the Greek language where *'sarcos'* refers to flesh and *'penia'* means loss (Physiopedia, 2019). Sarcopenia is characterized by loss of muscle energy, accompanied by the eventual reduction in muscle functionalities.

People with sarcopenia have reduced numbers of satellite cells. These cells are highly involved in the regeneration and repair of muscle cells, both of which lead to muscle growth (Physiopedia, 2019). This partly explains why the loss of lean body mass occurs as you age.

Coordination of muscle movement takes place in the brain. The changes that your muscles and joints undergo as you age affect your brain's ability to coordinate movements. As a result, you will feel weak, and your speed of movement is impeded. Let's discuss more on the changes that take place in the muscles as humans age.

Reduced Muscle Mass

Aging is usually characterized by atrophy. This is a scenario where muscle tissue is lost, leading to reduced lean body mass, which subsequently reduces function. Worse still, losing about 40% of lean mass has fatal consequences in your body. It is thought that genes might have something to do with the changes that take place in the muscles as people age (MedlinePlus, 2017). They determine the rate at which this process happens. Muscle changes tend to take place earlier in men than it does in women.

In older individuals, especially those above 50 years old, the lost muscle tissue is replaced by increased fat mass. These structures are, unfortunately, non-contractile. This decrease in muscle mass, alongside the accumulation of fat tissue reduces flexibility and impedes your movement. Please note this change in muscle mass was observed in the lower limbs of adults through a scientific research study (Henwood, 2008).

Another change that is worth mentioning is the deposition of an age-related pigment that is known as lipofuscin, in the muscle tissue. This pigment brings about a variety of changes, including the shrinking of muscle fibers and the slower replacement of muscle tissue. In cases where the muscle tissue is replaced, this happens with tough fibrous tissue. This causes body parts to appear bony and thin, especially the hands. The muscles become less able to contract, so they are less toned.

Lower Muscle Strength

Your muscles are powered by what is known as muscle fibers. These fibers power your movements and other activities that you might engage in. Even your day-to-day activities and chores are made possible by the existence of these fibers in your muscles. Now, as you continue to age, these fibers are reduced significantly and because of this, your muscle strength is also reduced. This explains why it becomes increasingly difficult for you to complete some tasks as you grow older. The same things that you once used to carry in your hands without any struggle might feel heavy for you as you age.

According to one study, changes that are related to strength reduction usually affect mobility, walking ability, upper extremity function, speed, as well as sit-to-stand and balance performance (Kahraman et al., 2019). The results that were presented from this study showed that significant changes in muscle fibers take place within one-year periods, in senior citizens.

Changes in muscle fibers occur in two major forms. These are

- **Changes in the size of the actual fibers:** Some muscle fibers reduce in their cross-sectional size as well as in their numbers. These changes negatively impact muscle strength as highlighted earlier.
- **Changes in size and number of motor units:** The proper functioning of the muscle fibers is enhanced by the presence of motor neurons. These are nerve cells that coordinate the functioning of the muscle fibers. In all human beings, loss of nerve supply and its restoration take place constantly. These two processes are referred to as denervation and reinnervation, respectively. In the elderly, denervation happens at a rate that is faster than that of reinnervation, thereby causing poor function of the muscle fibers.

Benefits of Stretching

In 2014, a study was done using seniors between the ages of 67-80 to examine the effects of stretching on muscle strength and flexibility. They were asked to participate in a static stretching program for about a year, and the exercises were to be done five times a week. After a year, tests were done on the participants, and the results showed that their flexibility went up by 31%, and muscle strength showed an increase of a 10-17% (Inami, 2014).

One of the effects of the physiological changes that happen when you age is a decrease in musculoskeletal flexibility. Your muscles become stiff, and daily activities become difficult to perform. By now, you are probably aware of the importance of including cardio, strength, and resistance training exercises in your lifestyle, but one area that is sometimes neglected and does not receive as much attention as it deserves is stretching.

Stretching is a type of physical activity whereby a specific muscle is stretched or flexed to tone the muscle and make it more elastic or flexible. There are many reasons why you should include stretching exercises in your fitness regimen:

- **It improves flexibility:** this is one of the key benefits of regular stretching. As you age, your muscles become shorter, tighter, and stiff, but stretching exercises or yoga can help with that. Stretching makes your muscles loose and limber, making everyday activities like getting out of bed, tying your shoes, and reaching for objects easier.
- **Increases blood circulation:** stretching encourages blood flow to your muscles and joints. This helps your muscles recover quickly after a workout and reduces muscle soreness. Plus, stretching can aid in the healing process of an existing injury, and reduce the risk of muscle strain and back pain.
- **Increases your range of motion:** stretching increases your range of motion by supporting your joints, ligaments, and tendons. Having an increased range of motion makes you agile and prevents you from sustaining injuries due to imbalance.
- **It improves your mood:** every day, we go through events that increase our stress levels and make it difficult for us to relax. When that stress builds, it may have a negative effect on our sleeping patterns and eating habits by causing unintentional weight loss or gain. When you are stressed, you get tired easily, and your body becomes open to both physical and

emotional health issues such as depression, heart problems, digestive issues, depression, and sometimes a weakened immune system. However, something as simple as stretching can change all that.

In 1993, a study published by the Department of Experimental Psychology at Oxford University determined that a simple 30-minute program combining both yoga and breathing exercises had a strong effect on both mental and physical energy, including a noted improvement in mood (Wood, 1993). Combined with the endorphins released when you work out, and controlled breathing, stretching exercises can put your body in a calm and relaxed state.

- **Helps in managing chronic health conditions:** when combined with exercise, stretching can reduce the risk of some chronic diseases like insomnia, anxiety, high blood pressure, and heart disease. They may also have therapeutic effects beneficial to your health.
- **Improves your posture:** having loose and flexible muscles prevents muscle imbalance, which is one of the common causes of poor posture. When you stretch, your core muscles are strengthened, supporting your body, and giving you the ability to stand straight and tall.

Stretching occasionally isn't going to automatically make you flexible or agile—it is going to take time and commitment before seeing any results. In addition, it is crucial to follow safety protocols and proper stretching techniques to remain safe and reap all the benefits of regular stretching.

Chapter 2:
Getting Started Safely

What to Know About Exercising as a Senior

If you were not as active as you would have liked throughout adulthood, you can't get into the habit of exercising regularly without ticking a few boxes first. Before starting your fitness journey, here are some things you should know.

1. **Talk to your doctor first:** You must talk to your doctor before starting any exercise program. Increasing your physical activity may affect the prescription and dosage of your medications. Your doctor may have to restrict you from doing some exercises at the beginning due to underlying health conditions.

It is necessary to talk to your doctor if:

- **You haven't been active for a while:** You may have cardiac complications or an increased risk of heart attack if you jump right in after being inactive for a long period of time. Your internal organs and joints will also need to be checked before exercising to reduce the risk of injuries.
- **You have arthritis:** Increased motion is a big help for people with arthritis because it strengthens the muscles surrounding the joints, but not all exercises can be performed if you are dealing with painful joints. So, you may need to consider different options, and choose those that will have less impact on your joints while pushing you towards your fitness goals. Your doctor or trainer can help determine the best exercises for you.
- **You've gone for surgery:** Doing strenuous exercises right after surgery puts a lot of pressure on your body, affecting its healing process. Pushing yourself too hard or getting into an exercise routine too soon after surgery can lead to complications such as infection, fluid buildup, swelling, wound separation, and bruising.

After giving your body some time to heal, your doctor may recommend basic physical therapy and low-impact exercises to get you moving again, in order to reduce the risk of complications and aid in your healing process. The intensity of the activities will gradually increase until your body is fully healed.

- **You've recently experienced a heart attack:** Exercising after a heart attack helps to reduce the possibility of having other heart complications, but you need to talk to your doctor about what type of exercises to do to recuperate faster, and determine the best time to start exercising again. Also, depending on the severity of the attack and the possibility of exercise increasing cardiac output, the doctor may be required to change your medications or dosages to suit your present health needs.
- **You have high blood pressure:** Being physically active is great for people with high blood pressure, but it may increase it, especially when you haven't been physically active. Ask your doctor about any restrictions that may apply, and the types of exercises you should focus on in order to reduce the risk of injuries, to ensure you get all the benefits of exercising.
- **You have diabetes:** Regular exercise affects how your body responds to insulin and can change your blood sugar levels. For instance, your blood sugar levels may drop after exercising, and pose health risks if it happens continuously.

Having a doctor guide you when exercising with Type I or Type II diabetes, or issues with blood sugar, provides that extra level of safety. You know what to look out for before and after exercising, and the steps to ensure that you are always healthy. For example, your doctor may advise that you check your blood sugar levels before and after exercising or have a snack after working out if your blood sugar level drops.

2. **Go slow but steady:** Going full speed ahead will only result in injury and setbacks and may cause you to stop working out altogether. Start with warmup exercises to get your body moving, and end every exercise session with a cooldown session. Also, get comfortable with low-intensity exercises, focusing on correct posture before increasing the intensity—once you've gotten comfortable with your form, you can take it up a notch. Also, pay attention to your surroundings for anything that can injure you, especially when exercising outside.

3. **Choose different exercises but make sure they are suitable for you:** the best part about starting your fitness journey is that there are a variety of exercises and workout programs to choose from. Include a mix of aerobics, strength training, balance, and stretching exercises, all with the right intensity to push you towards your goals. If you find it

difficult to do a specific fitness program, remember that it was made to fit you, and not the other way around. Put it aside, start with something easier, and go back to it when you can handle the program.

4. **Always remain hydrated:** committing to regular exercise means you must focus on eating well-balanced meals with just enough calories to fuel your body. Also, always have a water bottle with you and make sure to drink water before, during, and after workouts, even when you don't feel thirsty.

Exercising regularly for the first time can seem a bit daunting but implementing these tips can make it easier and encourage you to keep pushing forward.

Warming Up

Warming up is an essential part of any exercise commitment. It is vital in several ways – even more so as you advance in age. It physically and mentally prepares you to begin any routine and helps you perform at your peak and finish a session strongly. An entire workout session could be wasted without first warming up as your body might not retain any gains. A session could also be swiftly ended by a sprain or strain if the body doesn't properly warm up before undertaking the exercise.

Stretching for flexibility in all your body parts is part of an ideal warm-up, but it takes more than stretching to warm up effectively; you must also engage your hearts and lungs to aid in readying your muscles and body. Two of the finest warm-ups you can engage in are taking a short walk and marching in line with exaggerated arm swings. If you cannot stand, a modification would be to sit up as straight as possible in a chair and perform the marching with your arms and legs. The movement will still wake the body up and promote positive circulation while seated.

To get in the workout mood, keep doing this for at least 10-15 minutes.

Let's look at some of the most effective warm-up exercises you can do as an older person. There are various types of warm-up exercises, such as seated exercises and sport-specific routines. There is at least one routine from each section, so experiment and find which type works best for you.

Shoulder Rolls

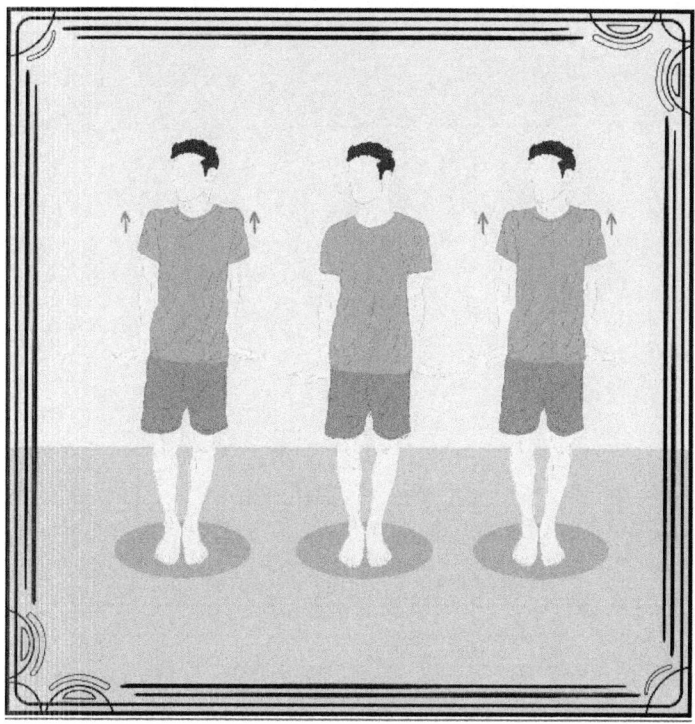

Benefits:

How often do you stroke your neck in the hopes of getting a massage? Several times a day, if you're like most people. Shoulder rolls can relieve discomfort and stress in your neck by allowing nutrient- and oxygen-rich blood to flow to those tight neck muscles.

Shoulder rolls should be included in any stretching practice for those who frequently battle stiff shoulders and back muscles. Shoulder rolls require you to place your body in posture-correct positions, which can help you improve your posture.

Because sedentary employment contributes to bad posture and associated aches and pains, shoulder rolls are an excellent stretching exercise for people who work desk jobs.

Steps:

1. Stand or sit tall with an open chest, neutral spine, and engaged core. Your shoulders should be kept back and down. Maintain a forward-looking position.
2. To begin, shrug your shoulders as high as you can toward your ears. Do not hunch your back, protrude your neck, or allow your shoulders to slump forward.
3. Squeeze your shoulder blades together and draw your shoulders back once you've shrugged as high as you can.
4. Pull your shoulders down by activating your mid-back.
5. Once you've reached the neutral starting posture, round your upper back slightly to press your shoulders forward while retaining a strong core.
6. Start a new shoulder roll by shrugging up again.

7. Perform 10 to 15 shoulder rolls, resting 30 seconds between sets. Three to five sets are a good goal.

Neck Stretches

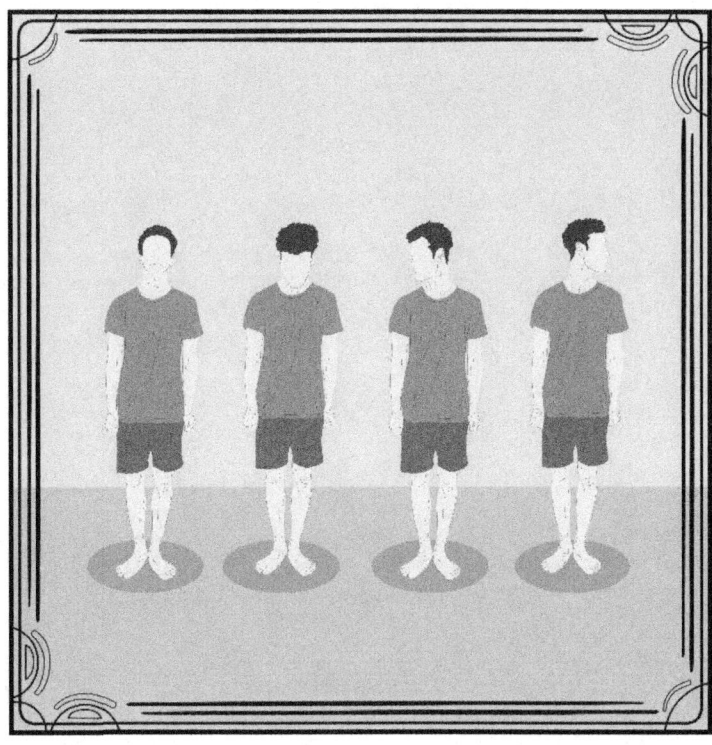

Benefits:

Neck stretches are like shoulder rolls in that they are very therapeutic. Neck stretches help to relieve tension in the neck and the muscles that support it.

By putting your neck through its full range of motion, you're preparing it to perform those movements again smoothly later.

These stretches should be used before any upper body movements. Surprisingly this is a good stretch to use before driving a car as it helps to warm the neck up in the case that you need to turn your head.

Steps:

1. Keep your arms by your sides while standing straight.
2. Bend your neck back as far as you feel comfortable. Looking up at the ceiling is ideal.
3. Lean forward until your eyes are on your feet. Tuck your chin into your chest as much as you can.
4. Do this a total of 10-15 times.
5. Bend your neck and look to the left, then to the right, with your torso remaining straight ahead.
6. Do this a few times more.
7. Make around ten circles in each direction with your head.

With the torso stationary, all your movements should be slow and controlled. You may perform these in a chair as well.

Lateral Arm Swings

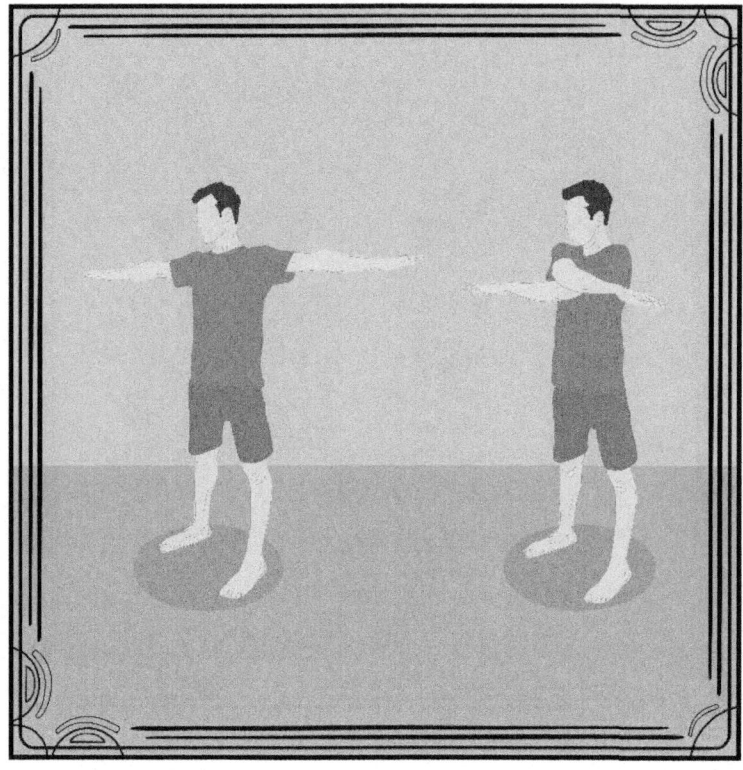

Benefits:

These should be used along with regular arm swings to increase circulation and warm up the upper body. This will help with motions that require you to raise your arms, reach across the body, or use your shoulder muscles.

Steps:

1. Stand tall and straighten your arms out to your sides with palms facing behind you.

2. Swing your straightened arms up and across each other, creating an "X" shape at chest level.

3. Return your arms to the original position by swinging them back down and behind your sides with palms facing the rear.

4. Repeat 15 times.

Wrist Circles

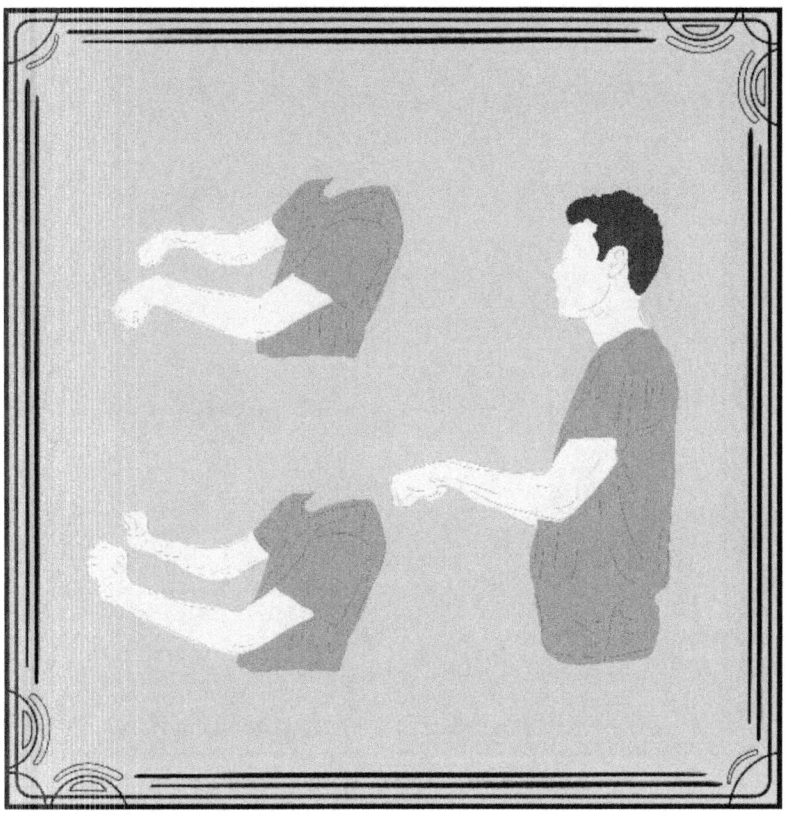

Benefits:

You spend a lot of time typing on a computer, texting on your phone, or simply just writing with a pen. This repetitive motion can often lead to awkward wrist placement that can cause discomfort or tightness in the wrists. You may even sleep in a way that keeps the wrist from moving very much or holds it in an awkward position overnight.

These will be useful for anyone performing workouts using their arms or attempting to grip something. These can help prevent wrist injuries while performing daily tasks as well.

Steps:

1. Stand tall and hold your arms outstretched in front of you. Maintain balance. Modification: If your arms can't be held outstretched, elbows can be kept at the sides and bent ninety degrees so that hands are kept straight in front of you. Perform the following steps from this position.

2. Without moving your arms, make outward circles with your wrists as if unwinding a spool of thread. Then repeat the motion making inward circles with your wrist as if winding a thread around a spool.

3. Perform eight outward circles and eight inward circles.

Leg Swings

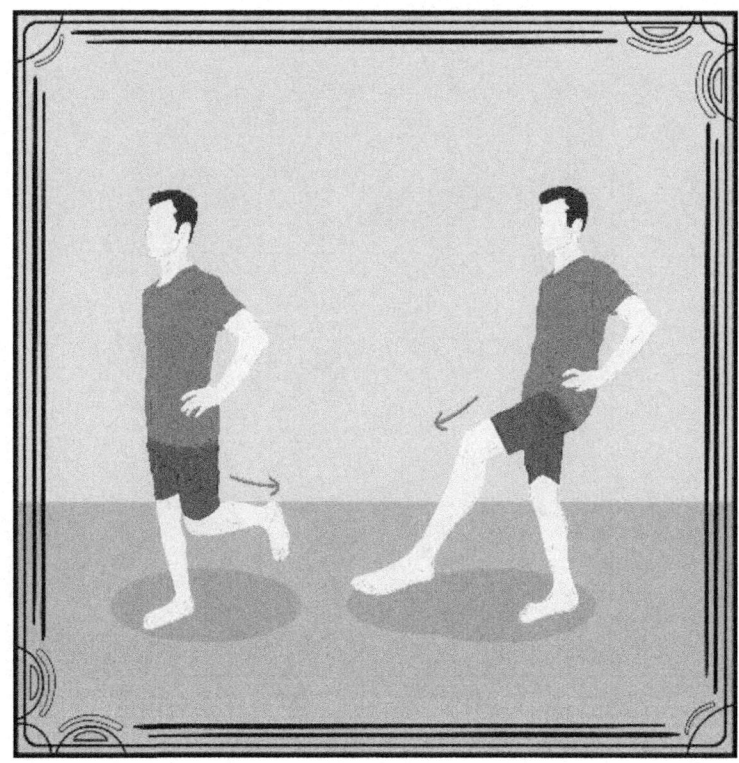

Benefits:

Leg swings are a warm-up exercise to target the hips. Using a chair or wall for support, you'll loosen up your hips, active the glutes, and stretch the muscles of the front and back of the thigh. These should be used before a walk, run, or lower body movements. They can also be used to loosen up the hips to aid in bending over with less tightness.

Steps:

1. Use your left hand to maintain equilibrium. Put your palm against a wall or grab the back of a table or chair.

2. Balance on the left leg and let the right leg hang loose

3. Swing your right leg forward and kick as high as possible without losing your balance or moving your left side.

4. After that, swing the leg back behind you. You won't be able to go back as far as you would like. Let the leg swing forward and backward comfortably without straining or forcing the motion.

5. Repeat this with the left leg.

6. Swing back and forth 10 times on each leg

Lateral Leg Swings

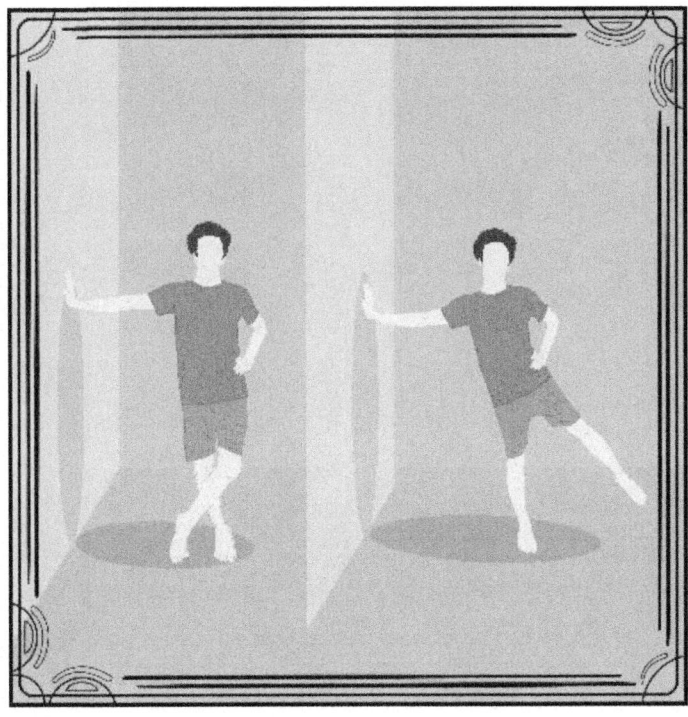

Benefits:

Lateral leg swings are all about activating the lower body. They put the hips through a full side-to-side range of motion, which can help improve balance and relieve hip tightness.

Use lateral leg swings to warm up the hips, glutes, and legs before a walk or performing lower body exercises. This warm-up can also help improve stability and maintain mobility when moving or shifting from side to side.

Steps:

These are like leg swings in that they continue to activate and loosen the hips and legs.

1. Brace yourself with one arm extended against a wall or standing holding a chair in front of you for support.

2. Stand tall with the left leg and let the right leg hang free.

3. Keeping the leg straight, swing the right leg across the body until it crosses over the left foot.

4. Swing the straight right leg from the crossed position out to the right as far as you comfortably can.

5. Repeat this motion going from left to right.

6. Complete this movement 10 times before switching to the other leg.

Ankle Circles from a Sitting Position

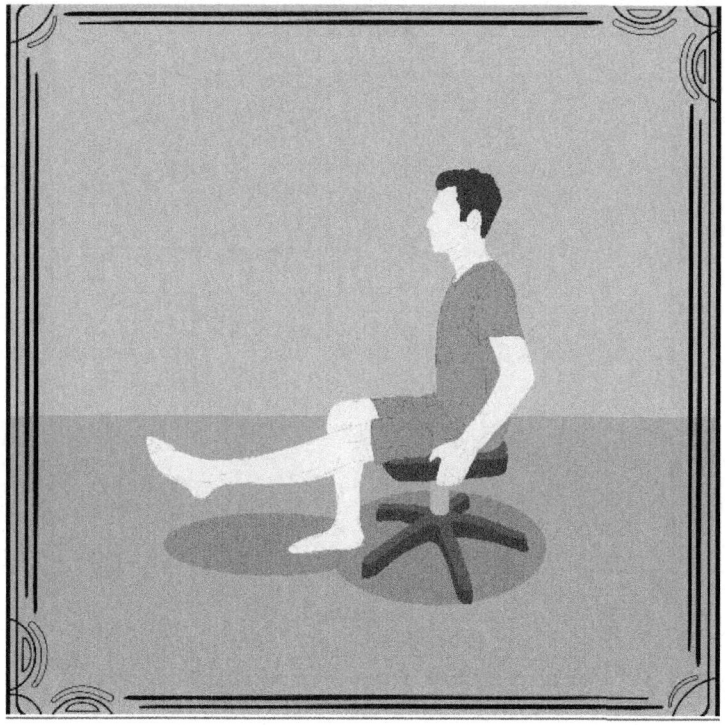

Benefits:

Ankle circles will help warm up your legs and feet. This warm-up can help prevent injury from rolling the ankle or tripping from the feet and ankles not being fully activated.

This is a good movement to use before a walk, lower body exercises, or even before getting out of bed first thing in the morning. Ankle circles can also help relieve tension in the shin. Shin splints (that cause pain in the shin) can occur from long periods of standing or repetitive movements that eventually aggravate the tendons and muscles.

Steps:

1. Take a deep breath and sit up straight.

2. Cross your right leg over your left leg or extend your right leg. It's fine to extend your leg straight out or bend your knee so that your foot is just off the ground when you extend. These two positions will have different sensations.

3. Rotate your ankles in a circular motion counterclockwise, maintaining as much stability as possible throughout the rest of your leg. These may feel jerky; as best you can, smooth them out. Then repeat the circles again in the other direction.

4. Repeat the process ten times more in the opposite direction.

For an added challenge, raise and rotate both ankles simultaneously.

Seated Hamstring Stretch

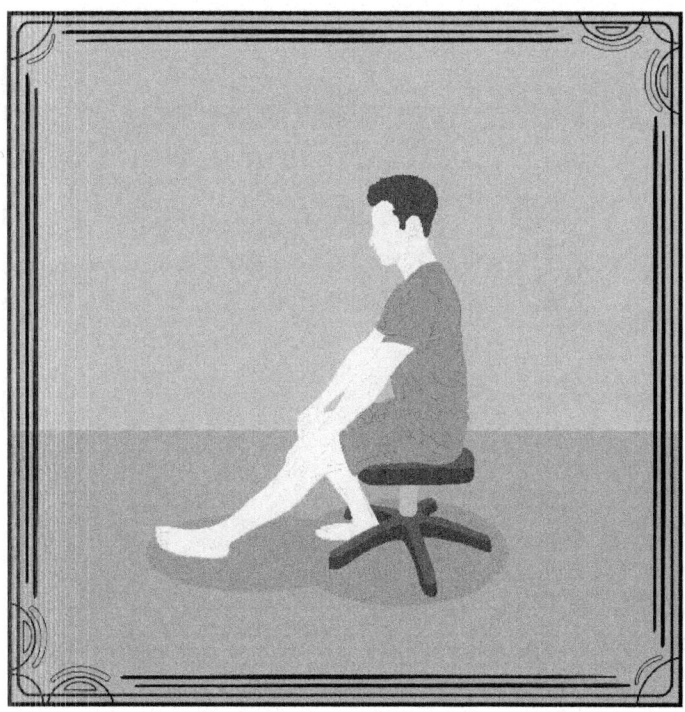

Benefits:

Your hips and knees are supported by strong, flexible hamstrings (on the back of the thigh), which help to prevent falls. They are a major source of power and are necessary for movement such as walking. Hamstrings can often become tight from lack of use, such as sitting or lying in the same position for long periods.

This exercise will loosen up tight hamstrings for more comfort and fluidity when walking. Perform this warm-up before lower body workouts or first thing in the morning upon sitting up in bed.

Steps:

1. Sit up straight in your chair or on the edge of the bed, feet flat on the floor and shoulder-width apart.
2. Extend your right leg, set your heel on the floor, and straighten your knee. (Your hands should be resting on your thighs.)
3. Slide your hands down your leg until a stretch is felt.
4. From the hips up, keep your back straight.
5. Allow your knee to bend slightly if it is stressed.
6. Maintain a 20-second hold. Deepening the stretch during the 20-second count is permissible but not required.
7. Switch sides and repeat.

Knee Bends

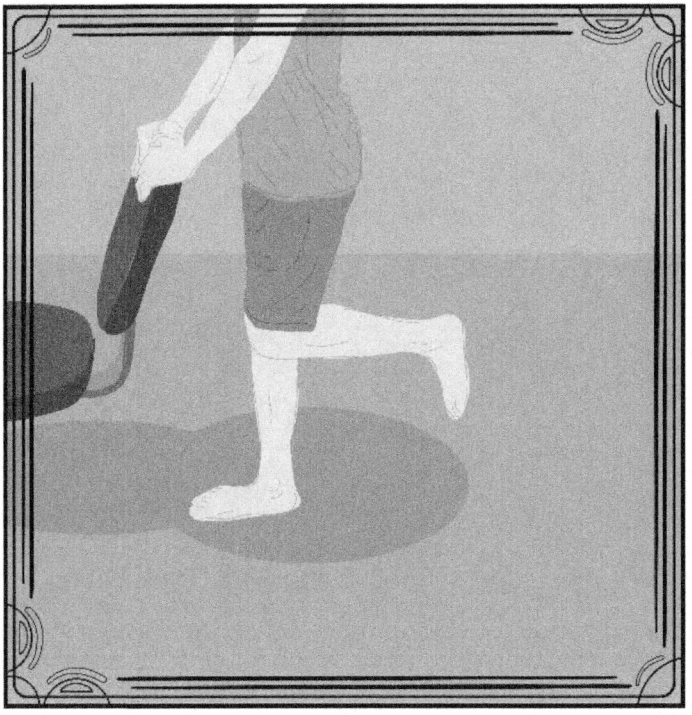

Benefits:

The knees are often a source of discomfort for many as we use them so often. They are sensitive joints, and the cushion within the joint degrades over time.

The muscles of the legs are often tight from sitting or lying in one position at night or during the day. The knee bend helps to warm up the muscles with a light stretch while moving the knee in its natural direction when bent.

Knee bends can help prime the knee joint while warming up the muscles of the leg. This can help prevent tightness or strain when performing lower body exercises, going for a walk, or just getting up and down out of a chair.

Steps:

1. Stand tall and bend one knee while keeping the other straight. This will lift your foot up off the ground and put it slightly behind you.

2. Once a stretch is felt in the thigh, return the foot to a natural standing position.

3. Repeat the movement ten times for each leg.

The Benefits of Warming Up

- **Heart Benefits**

The purpose of a warm-up is to get your cardiovascular system ready for a workout; your muscles will contract more fiercely and relax more quickly. This increase in heart rate improves the body's ability for strength and quickness. The heart also responds to warm-up movements by pumping more blood more quickly. Warming up your cardiovascular system makes it easier to meet the higher demands of a workout and prevents a blood pressure surge or feelings of unsteadiness from beginning too abruptly.

- **Increases The Safety Of The Workout**

Your brain and body must operate in unison for a workout to be successful and safe. Your nervous system needs to adjust to the change in activity and strain you'll be putting on the body during exercise. Warming up informs your body that it must prepare for a more strenuous activity than what it was doing previously, making your workouts safer and more efficient.

- **Helps To Raise Body Temperature**

When your body's temperature is slightly raised, it performs better. In the morning, warming up helps increase your body temperature, allowing you to notice a minor boost in performance. Getting the body "warm" means increased circulation and activation of muscles. Warming up before exercise aids in calorie burn as well. Getting into the "zone" with increased heart rate, blood flow, and maybe even working up a little sweat heats up and primes the body.

- **Increases Muscle Pliability And Oxygen Delivery**

Warming up increases your blood flow and muscular flexibility. When your muscles have been through their range of motion or activated with a warm-up, they are less likely to be surprised. When a muscle is surprised by a movement in a workout, it could result in an injury such as a pulled muscle. Warming up improves your body's ability to provide oxygen and nutrients to functioning muscles, allowing them to perform better.

- **Improves Cohesion**

Your nervous system communicates with muscles more effectively when it is adequately prepared. Your body responds with quicker reaction times and swifter motions when the nerve-to-muscle pathways communicate clearly. Warming up before exercise can improve exercise performance and allow for more difficult sessions with less risk of injury.

- **Increases Mental Acuity**

Stressed seniors are less likely to do well during their workouts. Stress causes them to become distracted and even slower. They also lose focus on the task at hand, become sloppy, and occasionally may be harmed. It's also a good idea to psychologically prepare for an exercise by clearing your thoughts, improving your attention, and evaluating your skills and approach; warming up before exercise provides mental preparation in addition to physical benefits.

- **Helps You Exercise Longer By Increasing Your Endurance**

Your body's capacity to exercise is harmed when lactic acid builds up in your blood. Lactic acid can build up faster in the bloodstream without a warm-up, making working out nearly impossible in the first few minutes. On the other hand, warming up can aid your body's energy systems to adapt to the increasing demands and reduce lactic acid accumulation, allowing you to exercise longer and harder.

- **Fires Up Metabolism And Energy Production**

During a warm-up, your body produces more hormones that regulate energy levels. More carbs and fatty acids are accessible for energy use due to this hormonal balance. Thus, warming up before exercise helps increase metabolism and enhances energy.

- **Increases Core Activation And Joint Stability**

Warming up your joints, particularly the hips, knees, ankles, and shoulders, helps improve your range of motion. A senior's capacity to move efficiently is limited by aging or less mobile joints, reducing power and causing one to slow down. Injuries to stiff joints are also common. Warming up the glutes, spine, abdominals, hip flexors, and back muscles helps your body stay solid and balanced during the workout.

- **Assists With Objections**

On days when you don't feel like exercising, a warm-up might help you get started. Warm-ups can be a fantastic motivator! A senior should warm up for at least 10 minutes.

Note: a warm-up can also be used to put your body that has been injured or sick to the test. Warming up can prepare the body for the day and help prevent the chances of injury for seniors.

Try to perform these stretches even on days when a workout doesn't seem likely.

How Long and Often Should You Warm up?

When it comes to warming up, how long should you spend? Professional athletes typically prepare for a game or competition for a long time. Tennis professionals, for example, practice for an hour before a match. Warming up muscles is not all professional athletes do; they're also practicing a set of moves (where they go through the motions of the movements they are about to perform for the sport).

Warm-ups for seniors should last at least 10-15 minutes and be performed right before exercise. Many warm-up exercises are beneficial to everyday activities and general health and, therefore, can be performed daily. Remember not to overdo your warm-up, and if you feel too tired, don't push yourself through further exercises.

Taking your time to engage in warm-up exercises before embarking on any of your choice workouts is a good practice with numerous benefits, especially for seniors. To aid in injury prevention and get your body and mind motivated and focused for exercise, it is highly recommended to perform warm-ups.

Chapter 3:
Essential Stretching Exercises

Neck

To regain the full range of motion in your neck, you need to target your muscles along all six planes of motion: forward flexion, backward extension, lateral flexion to the sides, and rotation to the sides. With greater mobility in your neck, you'll also enjoy deeper, more restful sleep as well as better overall function for longer periods of time.

Neck Flexion

Affected Areas:

- Back of the neck: levator scapula, splenius capitis
- Upper back: upper trapezius

Good For:

This is a wonderful stress reducer that is effective in relaxing the neck muscles that are most often impacted by chronic tension.

Level Up:

When your neck is fully flexed, gently rotate your chin first to your left, then to your right to activate additional muscle fibers adjacent to the targeted muscles.

Remember:

Take this stretch with you on the road. If you travel often for work and are prone to getting a stiff neck, try some neck flexion stretches to relieve the tension.

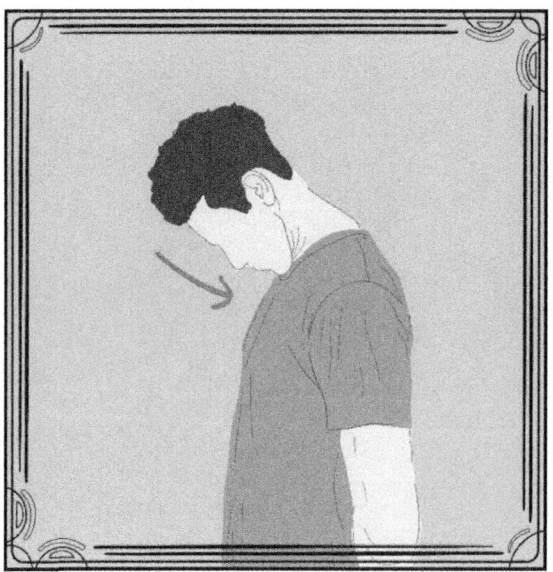

Instructions:

1. Stand in a neutral position with your feet shoulder-width apart or sit up straight in a chair with your hands loosely at your sides.

2. Inhale deeply to prepare, lengthen your spine, and loosen your shoulders.

3. As you slowly exhale, tilt your head downward, then try to touch your chin to your chest.

4. Hold for 15 seconds, continuing to breathe, and slowly return to the neutral position.

5. Perform three repetitions.

Neck Flexion Assisted

Affected Areas:

- Back of the neck: levator scapula, splenius capitis
- Upper back: upper and middle trapezius

Good For:

This stress-prone area sometimes needs a little extra work to improve the range of motion in your neck and increase the blood flow—both arterial and venous. By applying gentle pressure with just your hands, you can greatly enhance the benefits of this stretch.

Level Up:

As you become more comfortable with this assisted stretch, add progressively more pressure to the top of your head and hold for up to 30 seconds.

Remember:

Continue to breathe throughout the stretch to ensure that oxygen is continuously flowing through your body. If you feel light-headed or dizzy during this stretch, take a break. Next time, reduce the amount of pressure you apply.

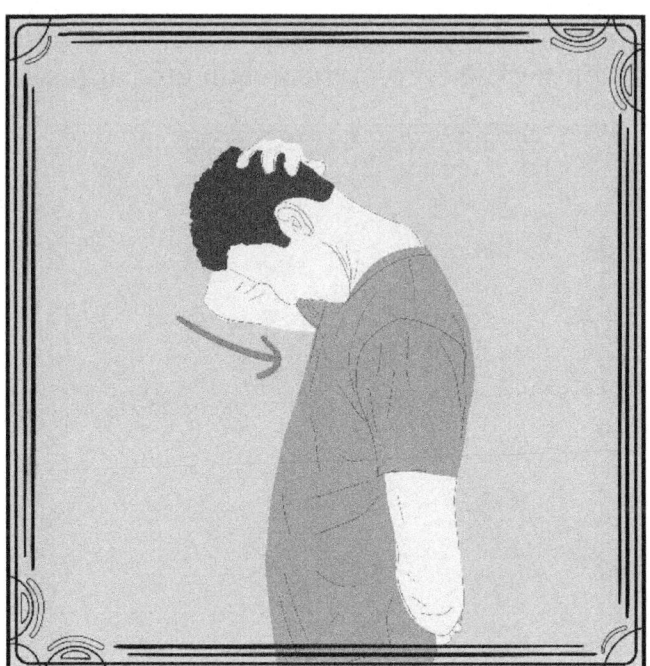

Instructions:

1. Stand in a neutral position with your feet shoulder-width apart or sit up straight in a chair with your hands loosely at your sides.
2. Inhale deeply to prepare, and place a hand on the back of your head.
3. As you slowly exhale, gently press your head forward and downward just slightly beyond your unassisted range.
4. Hold for 15 seconds, and return to the neutral position.
5. Perform three repetitions.

Neck Extension

Affected Areas:

- Front of neck: platysma, sternocleidomastoid

Good For:

Modern-day devices such as cell phones, tablets, and laptop computers all require you to constantly look down, flexing your neck muscles. Prolonged habitual use of these devices can cause the cervical flexion muscles to become shorter, stronger, and tighter. This neck extension stretch offers the perfect movement to combat neck strain and rebalance the mobility in your neck.

Level Up:

Engage additional neck muscles by adding a twist. As you perform the exercise, slowly and gently rotate your chin to your right and hold for five seconds. Rotate to your left and hold for another five seconds.

Remember:

Be sure to keep your back straight and your shoulders down while performing this stretch so you don't cause undue strain in your neck. Never let the weight of your head fall back quickly.

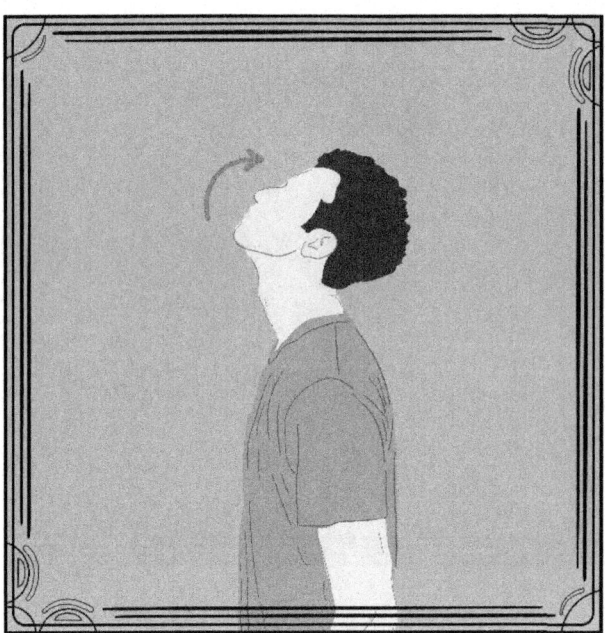

Instructions:

1. Stand in a neutral position with your feet shoulder-width apart or sit up straight in a chair with your hands loosely at your sides.
2. Inhale deeply to prepare.
3. Slowly exhale as you lift your chin and extend your head backward.
4. Hold for 15 seconds, continuing to breathe, and slowly return to the neutral position.
5. Perform three repetitions.

Neck Extension Assisted

Affected Areas:

- Front of neck: platysma, sternocleidomastoid

Good For:

If you tend to sleep on your back with multiple pillows beneath your head, this stretch can help counteract some of the muscle imbalance you may have in your neck. This is an excellent stretch for anyone with a forward head posture.

Level Up:

To target more muscles fibers in the affected area, gently and smoothly rotate your chin to your right side and hold for five seconds. Then rotate your chin to the left and hold for another five seconds.

Remember:

Alternate the supporting hand with each repetition for a more balanced stretch through your neck. Go slow with this stretch so you don't strain your neck or shoulders.

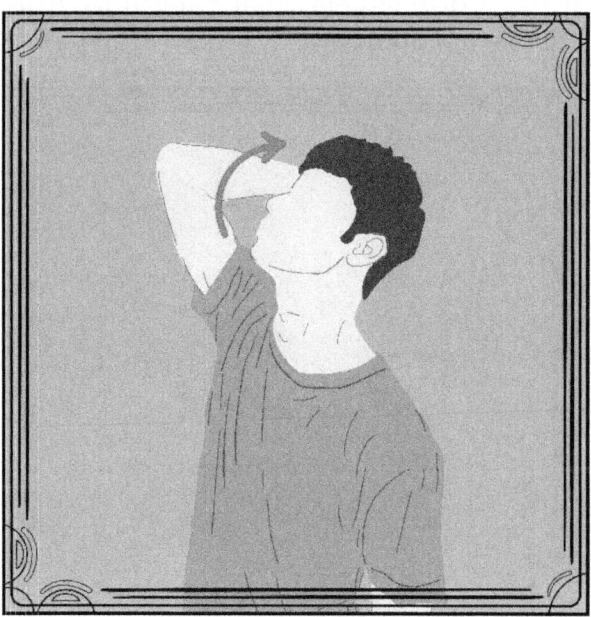

Instructions:

1. Stand in a neutral position with your feet shoulder-width apart or sit up straight in a chair with your hands loosely at your sides.
2. Inhale deeply to prepare, and place a hand on your forehead.
3. Slowly exhale as you lift your chin and gently push your head backward, slightly beyond the point of your unassisted neck extension.
4. Hold for 15 to 20 seconds, continuing to breathe, and slowly return to the neutral position.
5. Perform three repetitions.

Neck Lateral Flexion

Affected Areas:

- Sides of neck: scalenes, levator scapula
- Upper back: upper trapezius

Good For:

If you tend to sleep on your side, especially if you prop up your head with pillows, you may be putting unnecessary stress on your neck. This lateral stretch is highly beneficial for easing tension in the muscles along the sides of your cervical spine.

Level Up:

Ramp up the intensity of this stretch by stabilizing your torso while sitting in a sturdy chair. Hold onto the edge of the left side of the chair while bending your head to the right. Hold for up to 15 seconds and repeat on the opposite side.

Remember:

Concentrate on making sure the movement is emanating only from your neck. Don't lift your shoulders or bend at the middle of your spine.

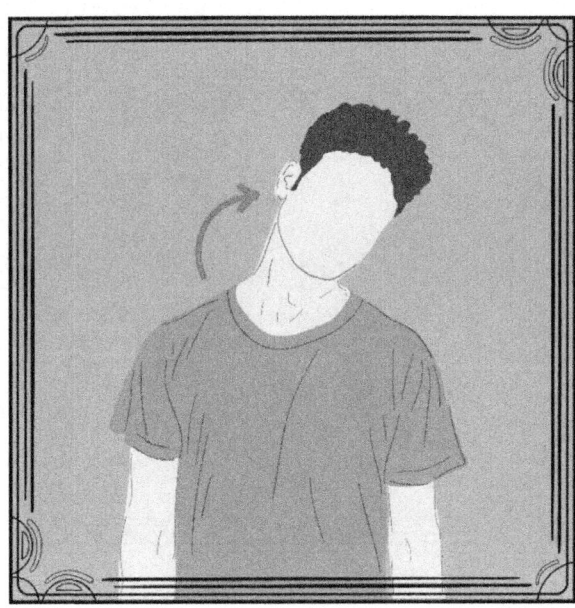

Instructions:

1. Stand in a neutral position with your feet shoulder-width apart or sit up straight in a chair with your hands loosely at your sides.
2. Inhale deeply to prepare.
3. Slowly exhale as you tilt your head to the right, as if to touch your ear to your shoulder.
4. Hold for 15 to 20 seconds, continuing to breathe, and return to the neutral position.
5. Repeat on the opposite side, and perform up to three times.

Neck Rotation

Affected Areas:

- Neck: sternocleidomastoid, levator scapula
- Upper back: trapezius

Good For:

Make the roads safer by making your neck more mobile! If you have difficulty looking over your shoulder to make safe turns in your car, this is the stretch for you.

Level Up:

When your neck is fully rotated in the basic rotation, gently lift your chin and hold for five seconds, then lower your chin and hold for another five seconds.

Remember:

Find a rhythm to your breathing. Inhale while you're in the neutral starting position and exhale as you begin the stretch. Most importantly, keep breathing deeply throughout the exercise.

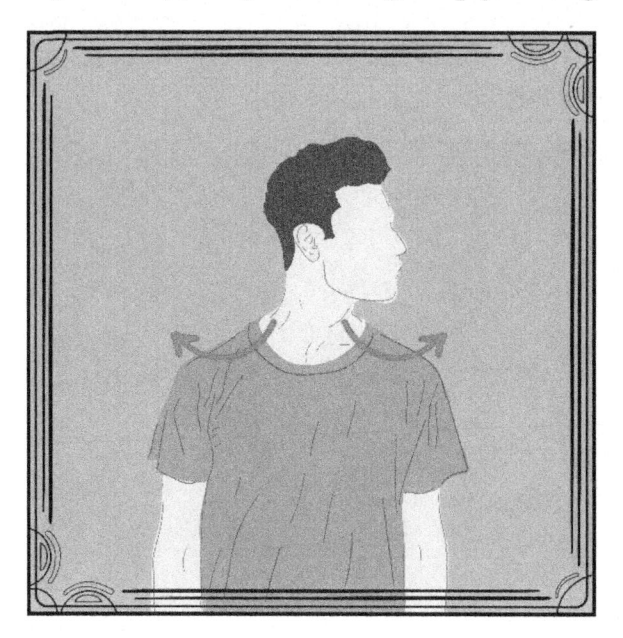

Instructions:

1. Stand in a neutral position with your feet shoulder-width apart or sit up straight in a chair with your hands loosely at your sides.
2. Inhale deeply to prepare as you lengthen your spine and drop your shoulders.
3. As you exhale, smoothly turn your head to the right and follow with your gaze over your shoulder.
4. Hold for 15 to 20 seconds, breathing deeply, and return to the neutral position.
5. Repeat on the opposite side, and perform three times.

Cervical Stars

Affected Areas:

- Entire neck: sternocleidomastoid, scalenes, levator scapula, semispinalis
- Upper back: trapezius

Good For:

Cervical Stars targets six planes of neck motion: flexing forward, extending backward, rotating left and right, and diagonal tilting to either side. This is a great exercise to perform for athletes to maintain the range of motion in their upper spine. Tennis players, golfers, and basketball players can benefit from this thorough neck stretch.

Level Up:

Gradually, intensify the stretch by holding for several seconds in each direction and using your hand to gently assist with the pressure.

Remember:

Always warm up your muscles before stretching. A hot shower in the morning is enough to get your blood flowing and get you ready for some exercise. Try waking up with a few reps of Cervical Stars while the hot water soothes your neck.

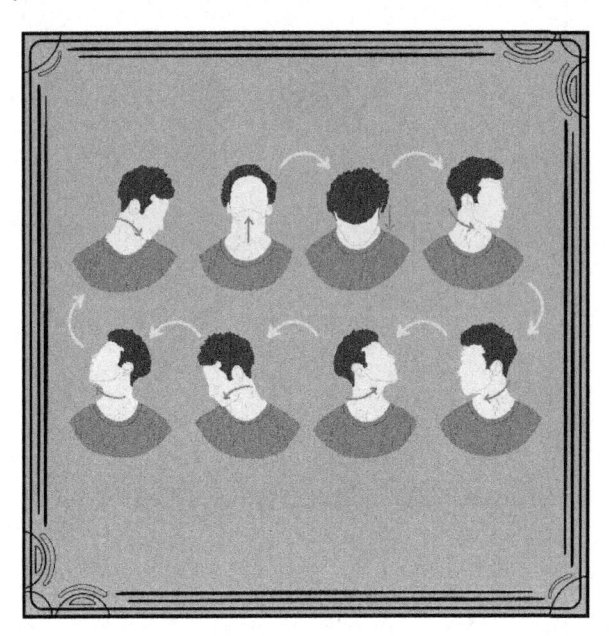

Instructions:

1. Stand in a neutral position with your feet shoulder-width apart or sit up straight in a chair with your hands loosely at your sides.

2. Imagine that there is a star shape in front of you with four intersecting lines: a vertical line, a horizontal line, and two diagonal lines.

3. Now imagine tracing those lines with the tip of your nose. Begin by slowly raising your chin up and lowering it toward your chest. Return to the neutral position.

4. Next gently turn your head to your left, then to your right. Return to neutral.

5. Raise your chin diagonally up and to your left, then down toward your right shoulder.

6. Finally raise your chin diagonally up and to your right, then down toward your left shoulder.

7. Return to the starting position, and repeat three times.

Back

Lower-back pain is one of the leading causes of work-related disabilities. Not only are the muscles of the back where we often carry stress, but they are also prone to injuries from lifting and twisting movements. Back stretches greatly improve the flexibility and resilience of your entire spine, from your neck to your tailbone.

Door-Assisted Side Bend

Affected Areas:

- Back: latissimus dorsi, teres major, teres minor, erector spinae
- Abdomen: abdominal obliques

Good For:

Many of us favor one side of our body and build tightness around overused muscles. This deep side bend lengthens the muscles in the middle of your back, one side at a time, so you can target the areas that need more flexibility.

Level Up:

Intensify the stretch by placing your hands higher on the doorframe. You'll engage more muscles all through the side of your body and along your spine.

Remember:

This side bend is a very effective, deep stretch that you can perform anywhere you find a door.

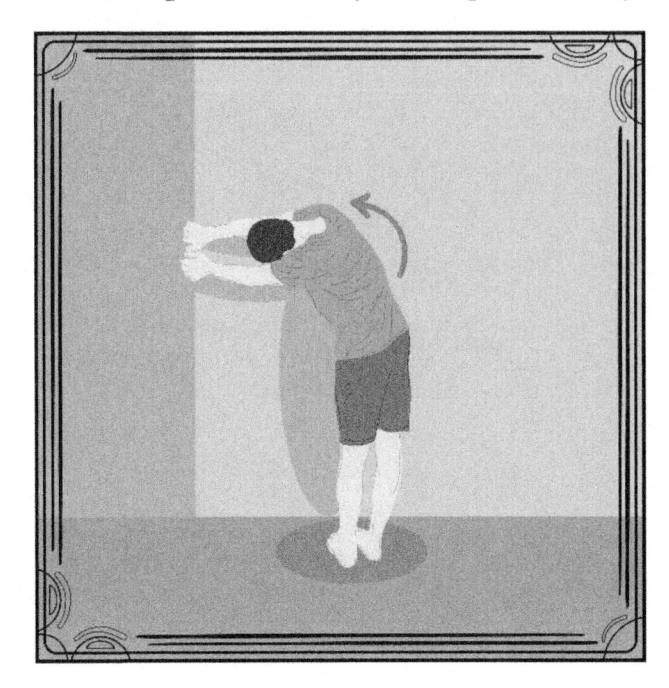

Instructions:

1. Stand straight with your feet together and about an arm's distance to the left of a doorframe.

2. Keeping your body facing forward, grab the edge of the doorframe with both hands, left over right, at about shoulder height.

3. Lean away from the doorframe, shifting your hips toward your left.

4. Hold for 30 to seconds and repeat three times per side.

Wall-Assisted Upper-Back Stretch

Affected Areas:

- Upper back: latissimus dorsi, trapezius
- Neck: levator scapula, spelenius capitus

Good For:

Poor posture and slouching can often lead to upper-back pain, as can prolonged hours sitting at a desk or driving a car. This simple stretch targets the muscles in your upper and middle back, lengthening the muscles along your spine and releasing pressure between your shoulder blades.

Level Up:

Engage additional muscles along the sides of your neck by turning your head slowly to your right and holding for five seconds. Repeat to the opposite side.

Remember:

Imagine someone is trying to pull you away from the wall. Keep your back straight and try to lengthen through your arms and your spine as you lower your head and shoulders.

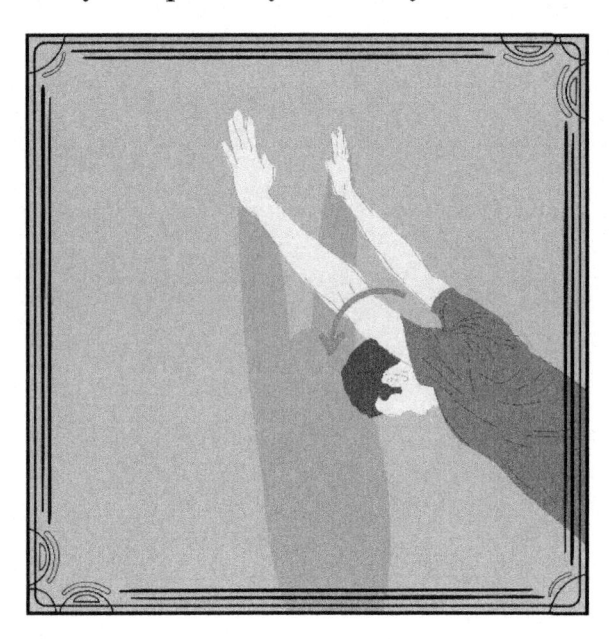

Instructions:

1. Stand facing a wall with your feet hip-width apart.
2. Press your palms into the wall at shoulder height.
3. Step about two feet away from the wall.
4. Turn your gaze down at your feet and pull your shoulders away from the wall while pressing your hands firmly into the wall.
5. Hold for 30 seconds and repeat three to four times.

Head-Tilted Forward Bend

Affected Areas:

- Upper back: trapezius
- Neck: levator scapula, semispinalis, spelenius capitus

Good For:

Although it's not quite an inversion, by bowing your head in this stretch, you can feel that it really gets your blood flowing. This gentle stretch also soothes tightness in your upper back and is a good exercise for relieving daily stress.

Level Up:

Clasp your hands behind your back, rounding your shoulders, and perform the exercise as above. You'll feel a slightly deeper stretch in your upper back.

Remember:

During dynamic exercises such as this one, find a rhythm to your breathing. Move smoothly with each breath, lowering your head on exhale and raising your head on inhale.

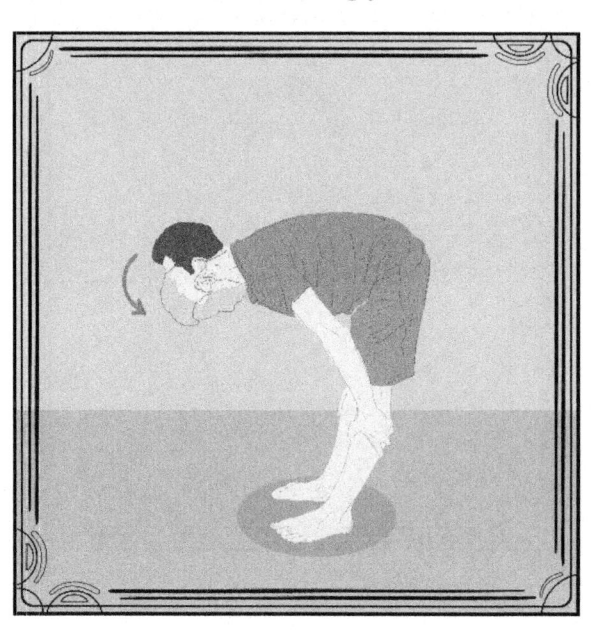

Instructions:

1. Stand straight with your feet hip-width apart.
2. Slowly bend forward from your hips and let your hands rest on your thighs just above your knees.
3. Inhale to prepare. Keeping your back straight, pull your shoulders down and back.
4. As you exhale, tilt your head downward, turning your gaze toward your knees.
5. Hold for a slow exhale, and slowly repeat the movement 10 to 20 times.

Bear Hug

Affected Areas:

- Upper back: rhomboids, trapezius
- Shoulders: posterior deltoid

Good For:

Nothing like a bear hug to release tension and tight knots between your shoulder blades. This stretch may also alleviate the stiffness associated with bursitis and frozen shoulder.

Level Up:

Perform the Bear Hug as above, except tilt your chin into your chest and hold for 20 seconds. This extra movement will further lengthen the muscles running along your upper back.

Remember:

When you're stuck on an airplane or a train and you feel tension building in your upper back, try this relaxing stretch to loosen up that space between your shoulder blades.

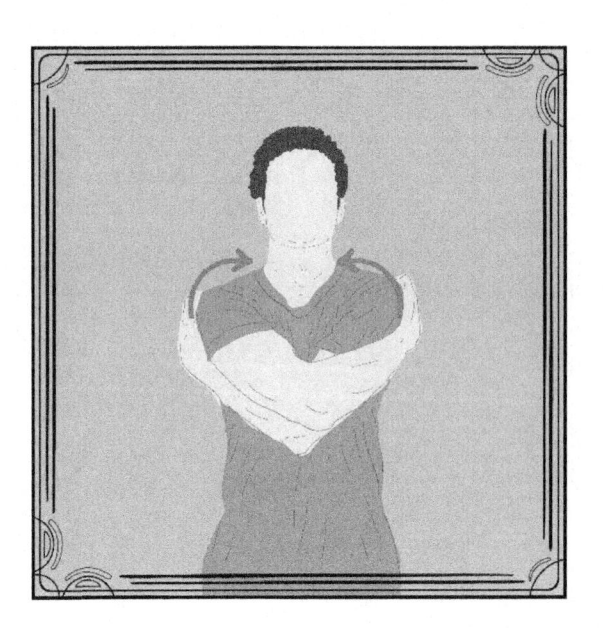

Instructions:

1. Stand straight in a comfortable stance.
2. Cross your arms in front of your chest, reaching your hands around your back and placing them on the opposite shoulder blade.
3. Press your hands into your shoulder blades and lift your elbows to shoulder height.
4. Pull your shoulders away from your body and hold for 20 to 30 seconds.
5. Release and cross your arms with the opposite arm on top and repeat twice per side.

Shoulders & Chest

Shoulders are often the repository of accumulated daily stress, tightening and rising up toward the ears. The chest, meanwhile, often becomes cramped and concave after spending hours working at a desk. The following stretches can help open both areas and restore proper posture.

Posterior Arm Cradle

Affected Areas:

- Front of shoulders: anterior deltoids
- Chest: pectorals

Good For:

This peaceful seated stretch eases strain in the front of your shoulders while opening your chest and lengthening your neck. If you're feeling stressed or simply longing to open the front of your body, this is the stretch for you.

Level Up:

For a deeper opening through your chest and lengthening along your spine, hold the stretch, and slowly tilt your head forward, bringing your chin into your chest. Slowly tilt your head backward, raising your forehead to the ceiling.

Remember:

This stretch can be done at home, in the office, or while standing, which makes it a great on-the-move option.

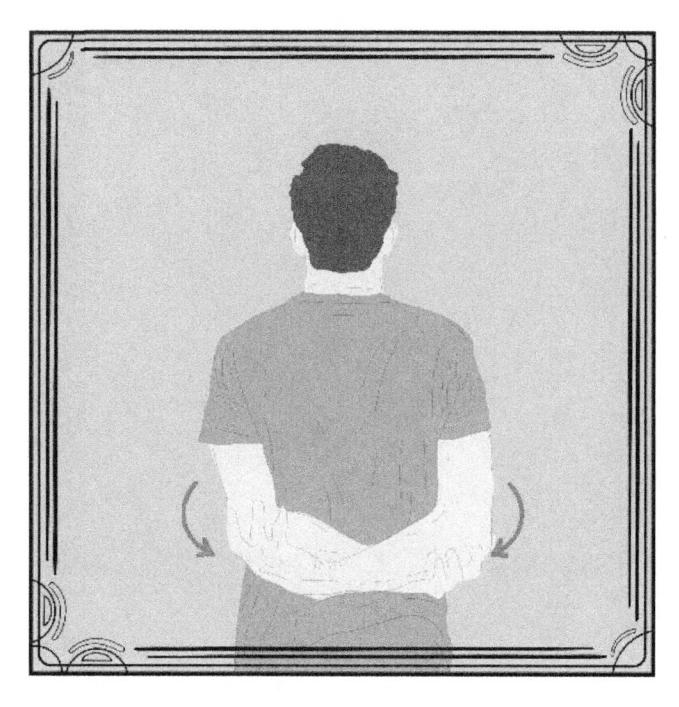

Instructions:

1. Find a comfortable place to sit, either on a floor or in a chair. Place your palms on your thighs and inhale.
2. Exhale as you push your shoulders down and roll them slightly back while lengthening your neck.
3. Gently bend your right arm behind your back and let it rest behind your hip. Bring your left hand behind your back to meet your right hand.
4. Slowly walk your hands in toward each other and up your forearms, settling at the opposite elbow.
5. Open your chest wide and breathe deeply and slowly for 30 to 45 seconds.

Arm Circles

Affected Areas:

- Shoulders: deltoids
- Upper back: trapezius, rhomboids

Rotator cuffs

Good For:

Arm circles provide an opportunity to get your energy flowing while expanding a full range of movement that begins from inside the shoulder rotators. If you feel tight in your neck and shoulders, this dynamic stretch will help release pent-up tension in those areas.

Level Up:

For an added challenge and more expansion through your chest, sweep your arms around in larger circles. When you're more advanced, try holding light weights or use weighted wrist cuffs.

Remember:

Proper breathing during this exercise will give you greater results. Although this is a dynamic stretch, keep your torso steady and control the movement to prevent pulling a muscle.

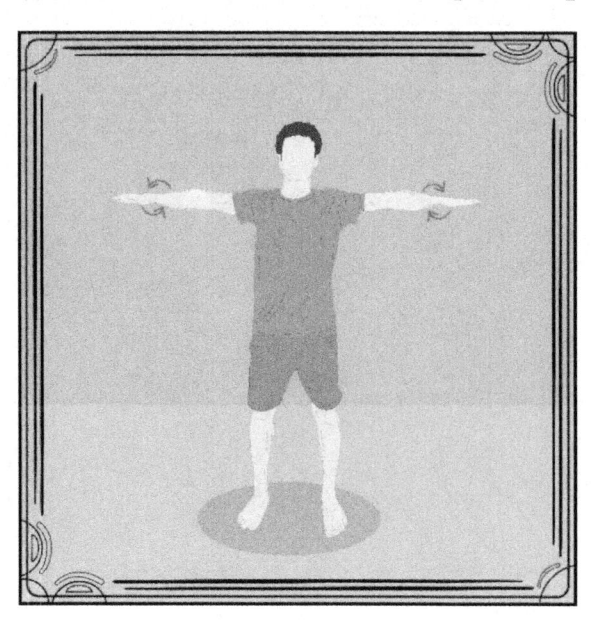

Instructions:

1. Start by positioning yourself with your feet spaced at hip-width and your arms relaxed, hanging down by your sides.
2. Effortlessly, extend your arms in a sweeping motion, moving them upward and outward while maintaining straight elbows.
3. Slowly rotate your arms forward and circle them down and around, forming small circles.
4. Repeat a series of five circles, and repeat in the opposite direction.

Wall-Assisted Chest Opener

Affected Areas:

- Chest: upper pectorals
- Front of shoulders: anterior deltoids

Good For:

This wall-assisted stretch opens your chest and lengthens the muscles that wrap around your shoulders. Weightlifters who build up their pecs would benefit from this soothing stretch. It also helps improve postural imbalances such as rounded or hunched shoulders.

Level Up:

For a more intense chest opener, place your left forearm on the wall slightly to your left. You'll feel a deeper stretch as you turn your body away from the wall. Gaze over your right shoulder to extend the stretch through your neck.

Remember:

Engage your core muscles and root down through your legs as you stand at the wall, so that your weight is fully supported from your center.

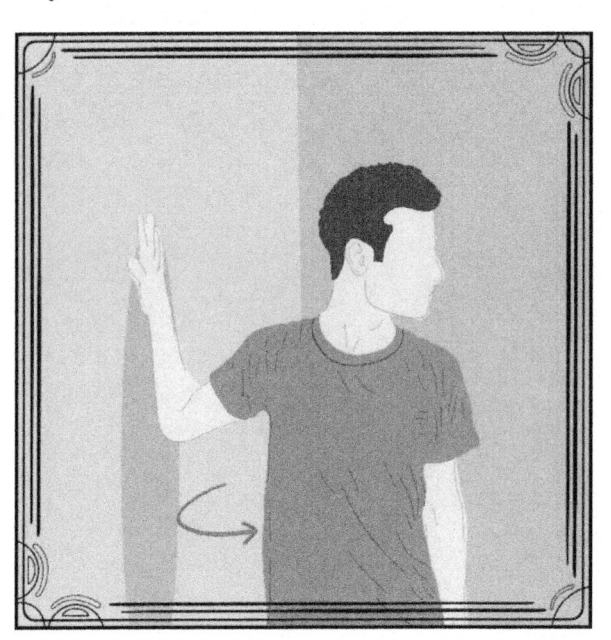

Instructions:

1. Stand facing a wall and about a foot away it with your feet hip-width apart.

2. Raise your left arm in front of you, bending your elbow to 90 degrees.

3. Rest your forearm and palm on the wall in front of you. Your elbow should be at the same height as your shoulder.

4. Shift your weight to your left foot as you step your right foot behind. Pivot your feet so that they are parallel to the wall and the left side of your body is facing the wall.

5. Press your left forearm into the wall as you turn your torso and head to your right.

6. Inhale and exhale deeply as you hold here for 15 to 30 seconds.

7. Switch sides and repeat three times.

Bent-Arm Fly

Affected Areas:

- Back of the shoulders: posterior deltoids
- Chest: pectorals
- Upper back: trapezius
- Upper arms: biceps

Good For:

The focus of this stretch is to align your hands, forearms, and biceps along the midline of your body. The opening and closing action of the movement shortens and expands your pectoral muscles while increasing mobility in your shoulders.

Level Up:

As your forearms touch, hold the position and slowly bow your head, tucking your chin into your chest between your arms. Inhale and exhale in this position for 15 to 30 seconds.

Remember:

Keep your elbows at shoulder height throughout the movement. If you are not able to touch your forearms together, simply bring your palms together at first, then gradually work toward pressing your forearms together.

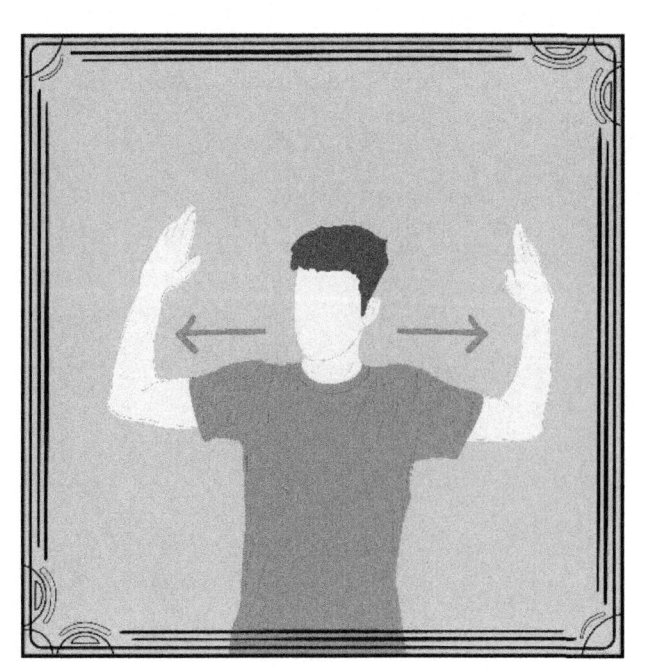

Instructions:

1. Stand tall with your feet hip-width apart.
2. Open your arms straight out to your sides with your palms facing forward.

3. Bend your elbows, making a right angle with each arm so your fingers point toward the ceiling, and inhale.
4. Exhale as you bring your arms forward, and press your forearms together near your face.
5. Inhale with your arms together, and exhale as you open your arms.
6. Repeat 10 times.

Elbow Circles

Affected Areas:

- Shoulders: deltoids
- Rotator cuffs
- Chest: pectorals
- Upper back: trapezius

Good For:

This stretch targets all the muscles of your shoulders and is great for improving your range of motion. The circular movement of this exercise provides a nice warm-up for your upper body and also lengthens the sides of your torso.

Level Up:

Intensify the stretch by performing wider circles and by pressing your elbows together at the beginning of the stretch. Try to keep your elbows in contact as they pass in front of your chest in either direction.

Remember:

Pay close attention to the range of movement in each of your shoulders as you perform these circles. Very often one shoulder is tighter than the other. Strive for symmetrical movements on either side.

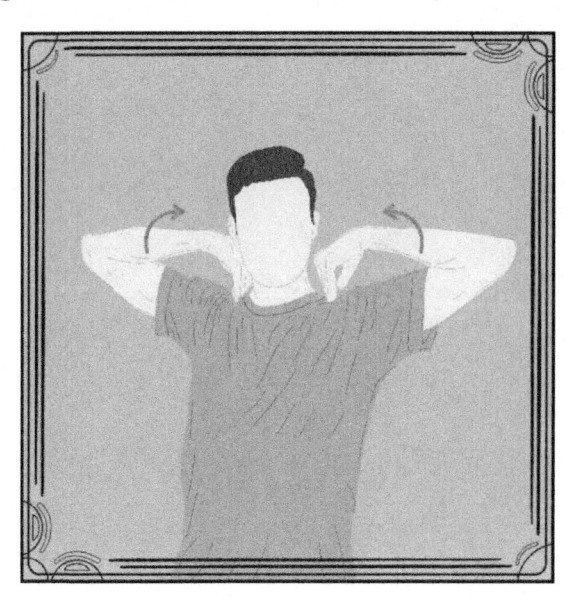

Instructions:

1. Touch your fingertips to the tops of your shoulders, and wing open your elbows to your sides.

2. Move both arms in unison as you trace your elbows in small circles, first to the front, then up and back, then down and around to the front.

3. Perform 10 circles and repeat in the opposite direction.

Extended Palm Press

Affected Areas:

- Upper back: trapezius
- Shoulders: deltoids
- Chest: pectorals
- Wrists

Good For:

Alleviate tension headaches, tight shoulders, and general stress that can affect your upper body. The Extended Palm Press helps ease tightness in your arms, neck, and shoulders as you move your hands along the vertical midline down the front of your body.

Level Up:

As your hands are interlaced at hip height, tilt your chin up slightly to feel more of a stretch along your chest. As you move your hands up above your head, allow your chin to fall into your chest to lengthen your upper-back muscles.

Remember:

If you are struggling with your balance during this stretch, have a seat and work through this stretch while sitting—it will be just as effective as if you were standing.

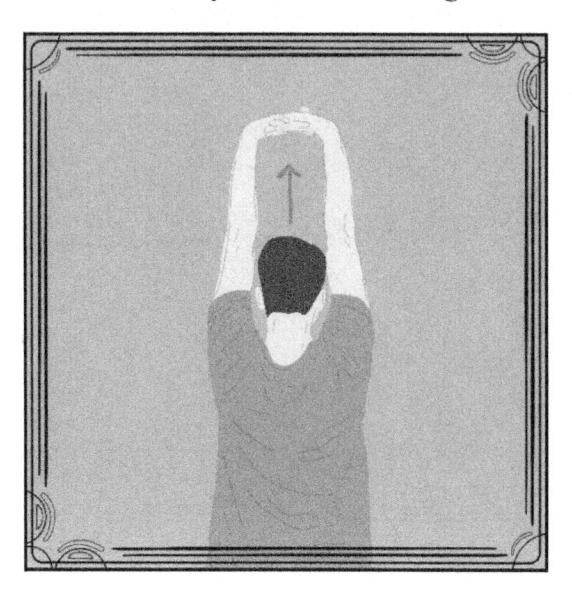

Instructions:

1. Stand in a neutral position with your feet shoulder-width apart or sit up straight in a chair with your hands loosely at your sides.
2. Inhale deeply to prepare.
3. Slowly exhale as you lift your chin and extend your head backward.
4. Hold for 15 seconds, continuing to breathe, and slowly return to the neutral position.
5. Perform three repetitions.

Crisscross Arms

Affected Areas:

- Chest: pectorals
- Shoulders: deltoids
- Upper back: trapezius

Good For:

The swing in this stretch activates your pectorals in two ways: by extension when opening your arms, and by contraction when crossing. If you're looking for an energetic release for your upper body, this is the move for you.

Level Up:

For added mobility in your shoulder joints, pitch forward from the waist and look down. Shake your arms out in front of your legs, and perform the stretch while bent over. Allow gravity to lengthen your arms out and away from your shoulders.

Remember:

Take your time as you swing through the crisscross movement. You really need only a little force to get a good stretch; less is definitely more with this exercise.

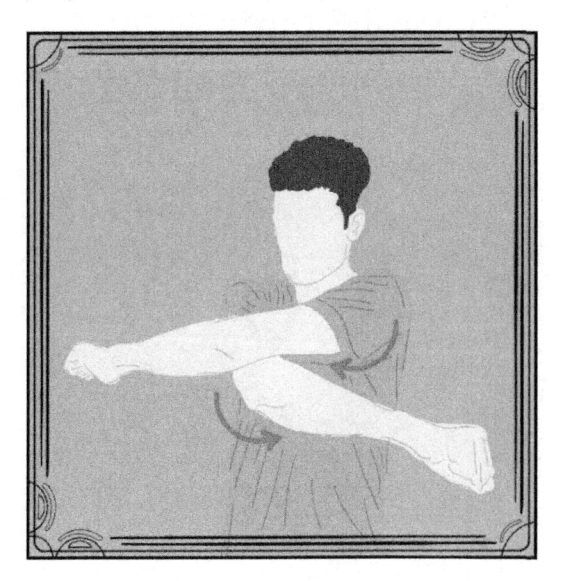

Instructions:

1. Start by shaking your arms out loosely in front of you, then down at your sides.
2. Give yourself a big hug with your right arm above your left arm. Inhale and exhale.
3. With a smooth, controlled movement, swing your arms wide open to your sides, and swing them back in across your chest, left arm over right.
4. Continue alternating your arm position as you swing open and close.
5. Continue for 30 to 60 seconds.

Shoulder Circles

Affected Areas:

- Upper back: trapezius
- Chest: pectorals
- Shoulders: deltoids

Good For:

Sometimes the smallest movements can have the greatest impact. When you have a moment of peace, close your eyes and allow this stretch to melt away pent-up tension in your upper body. Perform these shoulder circles as big or as small as you'd like.

Level Up:

Expand the stretch into the sides of your neck by isolating one shoulder at a time. Lean your right ear toward your right shoulder as you circle your left shoulder. Then lean your left ear toward your left shoulder as you circle your right shoulder.

Remember:

This is a very effective stress-relieving stretch that can be done multiple times a day. And you can take it with you anywhere you go.

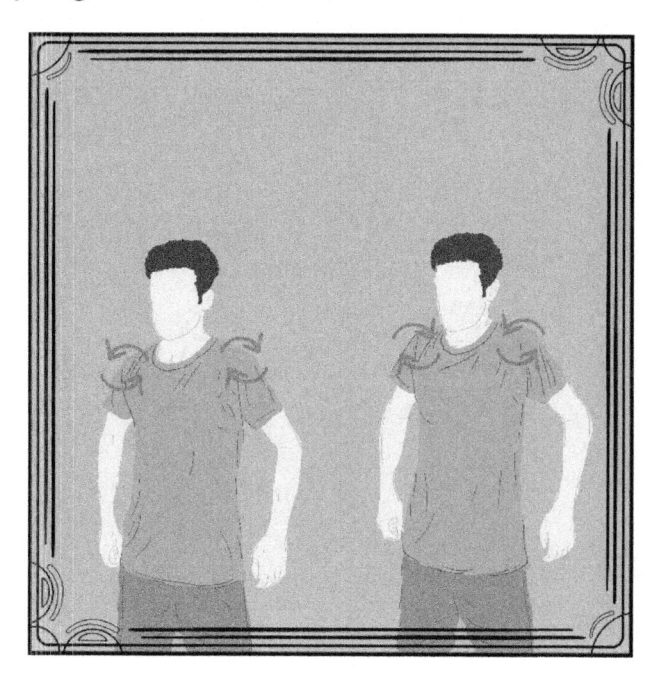

Instructions:

1. Stand straight with your feet about hip-width apart. Allow you arms to dangle loosely at your sides.
2. Breathe in, and focus your attention on your shoulders.

3. Shrug your shoulders up toward your ears, and circle them back and around to the front.
4. Repeat 10 times in each direction.

Arms, Wrists, & Hands

The arms, along with the wrists and hands, are the versatile workhorses of the body—performing feats of physical strength and detailed maneuvers. Arm stretches also benefit the delicate mechanisms of the wrists and hands by strengthening them against injury and relieving stiffness and pain.

Wall-Assisted Bicep Stretch

Affected Areas:

- Shoulders: deltoids
- Chest: upper pectorals
- Upper arms: biceps
- Forearms: brachialis

Good For:

This simple wall-assisted stretch lengthens the muscles along your chest, down your arms, and into your wrists. Find soothing relief from tight chest muscles and stiff shoulders and arms.

Level Up:

For a more intense opening along the back of your neck, slowly turn your head away from the wall to look toward the opposite shoulder.

Remember:

Root down through your legs and engage your core muscles so that your weight is fully supported from your center. Try not to tense up your shoulders.

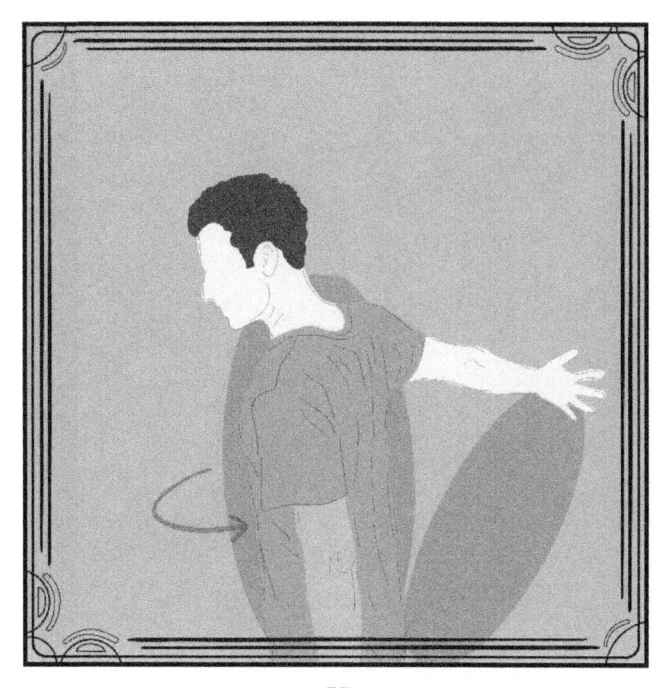

Instructions:

1. Stand with your right side about a foot away from a wall.

2. Step your left foot forward into an open stance.

3. Extend your right arm to shoulder height, and rest the palm of your hand on the wall above you.

4. Keeping contact with the wall, allow your right arm to slowly circle back and down behind you, bringing your hand to rest just below shoulder height.

5. Open your chest and slightly bend your left knee, shifting your weight several inches forward.

6. Inhale and exhale deeply as you hold here for 15 to 30 seconds.

7. Switch sides and repeat three times on each arm.

Tricep Stretch

Affected Areas:

- Upper arms: triceps, biceps
- Shoulders: deltoids

Good For:

Counterbalance the downward pull of gravity on your arms by lifting your arms overhead and lengthening the sides of your body. You'll be able to loosen the area along the back of your arms as well as find some solace from tight shoulders.

Level Up:

Throw in a towel to ramp up this stretch. Grab one end of a rolled-up towel with your raised arm. Bring your opposite hand to your lower back and gently pull on the towel for 15 to 30 seconds.

Remember:

Try to engage your core muscles and open your chest as you perform this exercise. Keep your back straight throughout.

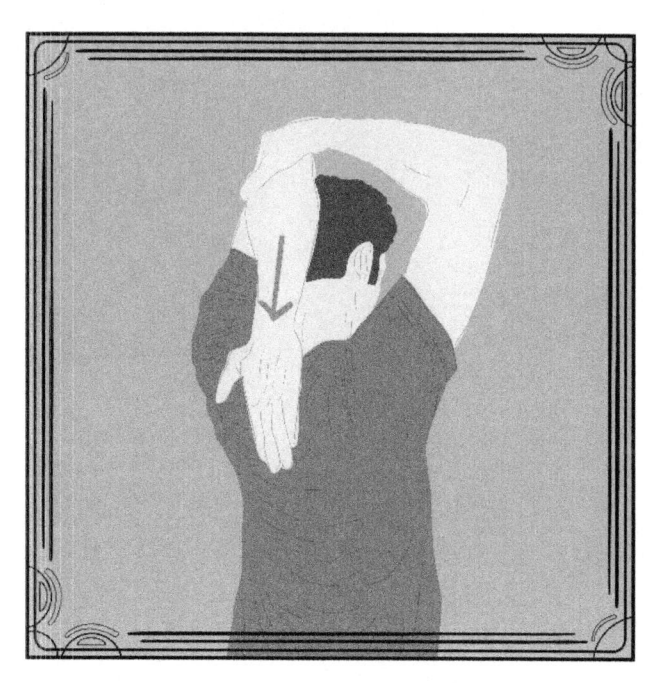

Instructions:

1. Find a comfortable stance or a supported seated position.
2. Raise your left arm straight up along your left ear.
3. Turn your arm inward so that your palm is facing behind you.
4. Bring your right hand up to support your left elbow as you slowly bend your left elbow, reaching your palm to the back of your left shoulder.

5. Use your right hand to gently press your left elbow up and back for a stretch. Hold for 20 seconds at the top of the move and breathe.
6. Repeat three to four times.

Wrist Flexion

Affected Areas:

- Upper arms: biceps
- Forearms: pronators, extensors, wrist flexors

Good For:

If your daily routine involves a lot of work with your hands or you have a hobby such as weight lifting, tennis, cooking, sewing, or gardening, this simple dynamic stretch will provide extensive relief through your wrists, forearms, and fingers.

Level Up:

Intensify the stretch by curling your extended fingers into a downward-facing fist. While keeping light pressure on the back of your wrist with your supporting hand, gently pull your fist down and away from your wrist.

Remember:

The shoulder of the extended arm will naturally want to lift, but try to keep both shoulders square and relaxed. Imagine pulling your shoulder blades down your back.

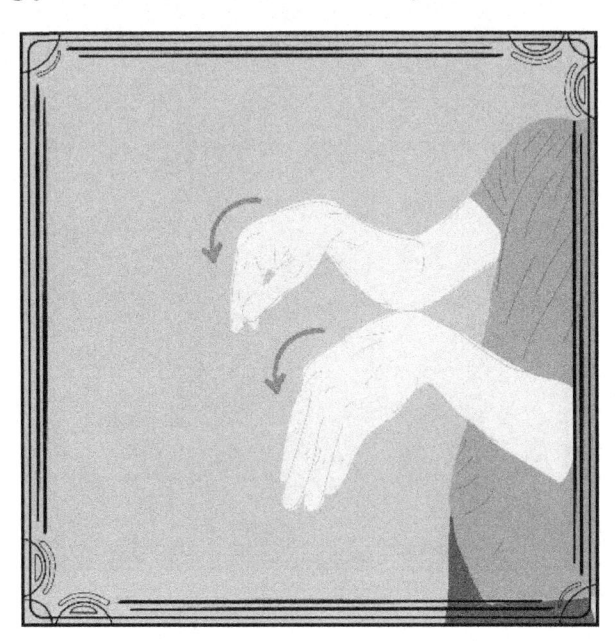

Instructions:

1. Begin either standing or seated, and extend your left arm straight out in front of you.
2. Press your left fingers and thumb together, and flex your wrist downward, pointing your fingers toward the floor.
3. With your right hand, gently press your left fingers bringing them closer in to your body.
4. Hold for 15 to 30 secs, and repeat three to four times.

Wall-Assisted Forearm Stretch

Affected Areas:

- Upper arms: biceps
- Forearms: pronators, extensors, wrist flexors

Good For:

This highly effective stretch calls for you to turn your arm outward, exposing your inner forearm up to the ceiling while bringing your wrist into full extension. With the support of the wall, this stretch is ideal for anyone who needs a little extra help with balance.

Level Up:

Tilt your head away from the wall to feel more lengthening through your upper arm, shoulder, and neck.

Remember:

Try to open your fingers as wide as you can while your palm is in contact with the wall. This will assure an even stretch through your hand and fingers.

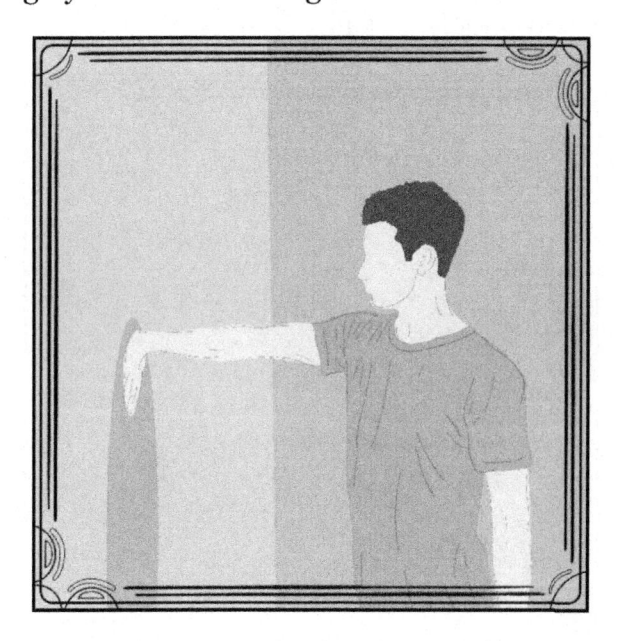

Instructions:

1. Stand with your right side positioned about arm's distance from a sturdy wall.
2. Bring your palm into contact with the wall, and spin your palm counterclockwise, pointing your fingers down toward the floor.
3. Press your palm into the wall by shifting your weight toward your arm.
4. Press your elbow up and open to the ceiling as you press your palm against the wall.
5. Hold for 15 to 20 seconds, and repeat on the opposite arm.
6. Perform three sets.

Prayer Hands

Affected Areas:

- Forearms: flexors, pronators, extensors
- Wrists

Good For:

Achieving the symmetry of this pose calls for you to focus on the midline of your body as you press your hands together and open the front of your chest. Prayer hands may help alleviate pain associated with ailments such as tennis elbow and arthritis.

Level Up:

When you're ready, advance to this dynamic variation. As you stretch through your arms, slowly extend your prayer hands above your head, keeping your palms pressed together, and slowly lower your hands back down toward the center of your chest. Repeat for up to 60 seconds.

Remember:

To achieve the ultimate symmetry of this stretch, be sure to form a straight line from elbow to elbow and along your forearms while keeping your palms pressed together.

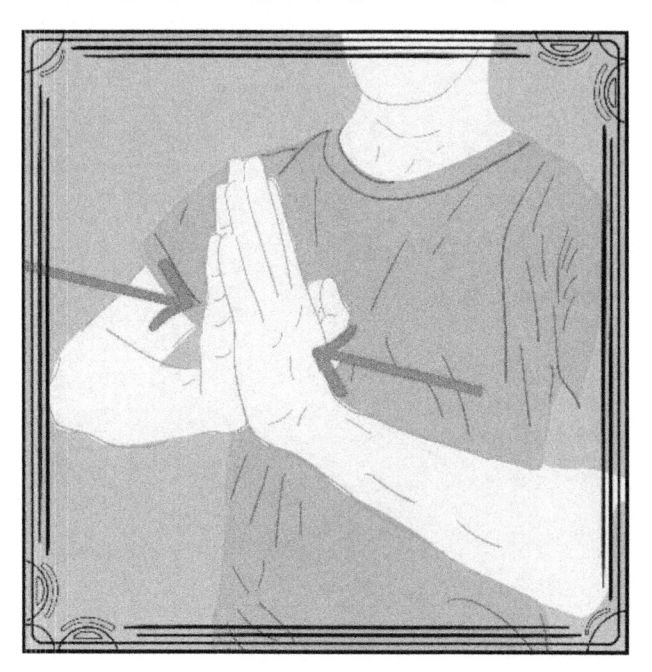

Instructions:

1. Begin in a comfortable position either standing or sitting.
2. Inhale and press your palms together in front of your chest, with your fingers touching your chin.

3. Exhale as you press the base of your palms, fingers, and thumbs firmly together and lower your hands toward your waist.

4. Hold for 15 to 30 seconds, and repeat three times.

Finger Stretch

Affected Areas:

- Forearms: flexors, pronators, wrist extensors

Hands

Fingers

Good For:

Hours of scrolling on your computer or texting on your phone can lead to overuse of your fingers, causing stiffness, tenderness, and pain in your arms, elbows, and wrists. Take some time to open up the spaces between your fingers with this simple stretch.

Level Up:

For an added stretch through your wrists, flip your hands over so that your palms are facing up. Now, curl your fingers into tight fists and hold for 10 seconds. Then slowly release your fists and open your hands. Wiggle your fingers and repeat three times.

Remember:

Your thumbs can easily become more immobile than your fingers, so pay attention to how you splay your hands open. Give extra attention to your thumbs, pulling them gently open and in toward each other.

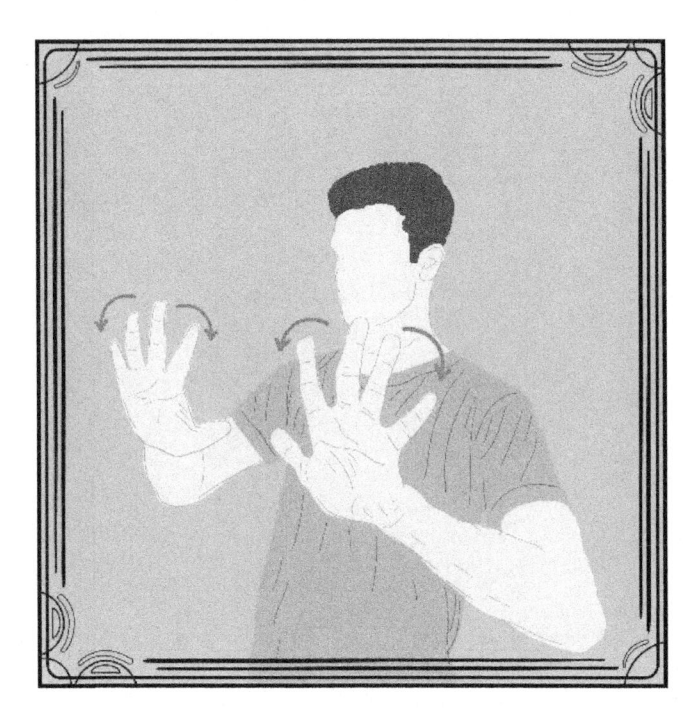

Instructions:

1. Choose a comfortable place where you can stand easily or can sit with support from a chair.

2. Extend your arms out in front of your chest, keeping your elbows slightly bent.

3. Press your fingers and thumbs together so that there's no space between them, and hold for five seconds.

4. Next splay your fingers wide open, creating a lot of space between them. Hold for five seconds.

5. Repeat five times.

Thumb Stretch

Affected Areas:

- Thumbs: flexors, extensors, pro nadirs

Good For:

Our hands get a workout all day long: We text, type, play musical instruments, and do various chores. Yet rarely do we take the time to pamper our tired hands and, in particular, our thumbs. These isolated stretches are most impactful when you're fully relaxed.

Level Up:

Turn this stretch into a dynamic exercise and rotate your thumb in circles with your opposite hand. Keep your palm steady as you move your thumb.

Remember:

This is a very soothing stretch that can be done seated, lying down, or standing. It is especially valuable because you can perform it anywhere you go.

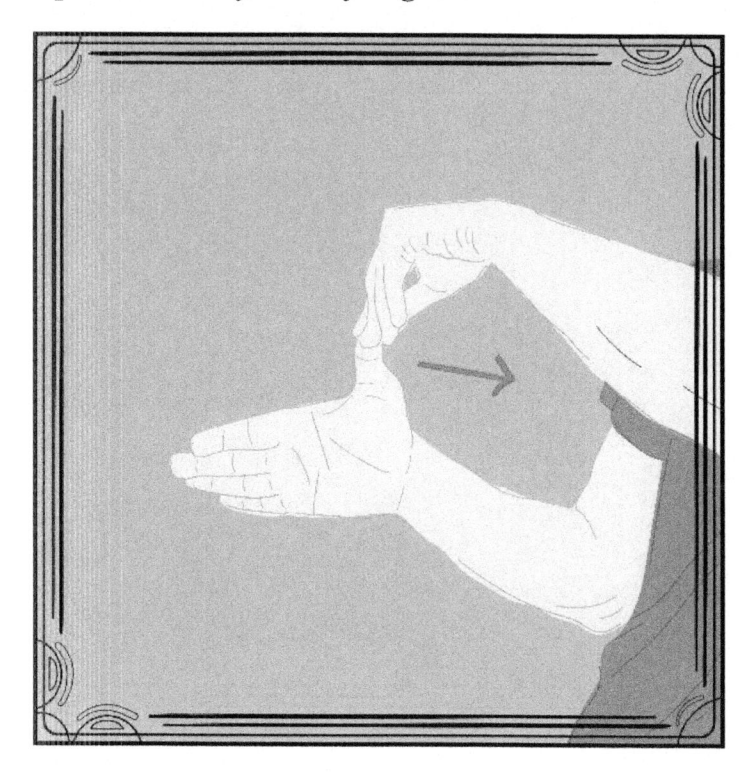

Instructions:

1. Find a comfortable place to sit.
2. Hold your right hand in front of your chest, with your palm facing your chest.

3. Wrap your left hand around your right thumb. Keeping your right hand in line with your forearm, push your thumb downward, and hold for 10 seconds.

4. Flex your wrist toward your chest. Push your thumb toward your forearm, and hold for 10 seconds.

5. Next, extend your wrist so your palm is perpendicular to your chest. Again push on your thumb, and hold for 10 seconds.

6. Repeat on the opposite hand.

Core & Hips

Core stretches benefit a group of critical muscles, toning your abdominals along the front and sides of your torso. These stretches improve your balance and sports performance. Hip stretches are also essential for maintaining proper balance and coordination. By performing core and hip stretches regularly, you'll improve the range of motion in your lower body and help protect against injuries.

Hip Twist

Affected Areas:

- Buttocks: gluteals
- Hip rotators: piriformis, quadratus femoris
- Abdomen: abdominal obliques, transverse abdominus

Good For:

Open those hard-to-reach muscles that wrap across your lower back and hips, and along the sides of your torso. The twisting movement of this stretch helps improve posture and lower-back pain.

Level Up:

Intensify this twisted movement by pushing down strongly into your right hand. Lift your core up and in, and straighten your left arm, reaching your left fingertips down to the floor.

Remember:

If you find it challenging to sit up straight through your lower spine in this pose, place a rolled-up towel, yoga block, or firm pillow under your hips for support.

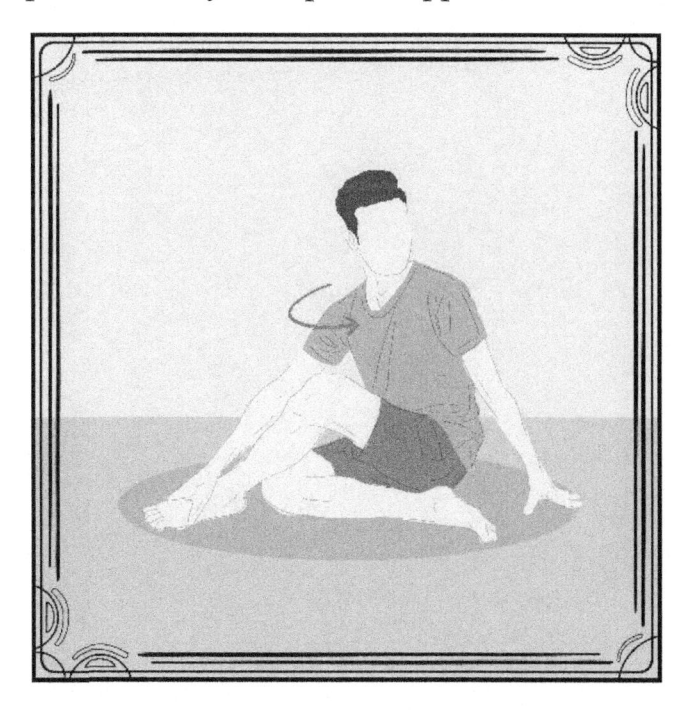

Instructions:

1. Sit with your legs extended in front of you.
2. Step your left foot over your right knee, and rest your left foot on the floor just outside your right knee.
3. Place your left hand on the floor near your left hip, and put weight on it for support.
4. Raise your right arm, pull in your abs, and root your left foot down. Lengthen through your spine as you twist your torso to your left.
5. Lower your right arm. Bend your right elbow, and place it on the outside of your left knee.
6. Push down into your left arm and twist your upper torso, turning your head to look to your left.
7. Hold for 20 to 30 seconds, and repeat three times on each side.

Triangle Pose

Affected Areas:

- Abdomen: abdominal obliques, transverse abdominus
- Back: erector spinae
- Inner thighs: adductors

Good For:

With its origins in yoga, the Triangle Pose offers a deep stretch along the back and front of your lower abdomen while lengthening the sides of your torso and back. This is a fantastic stretch if you're experiencing stiffness through your lower back and hips.

Level Up:

For an advanced stretch, lower your hand from your ankle down to the floor in front of your foot, and try to place your palm on the floor. Push forward with your pelvis and lengthen through your arms, forming a straight line from hand to hand.

Remember:

If this stretch is too challenging for you at first, you may place your hand on your shin rather than your ankle. Find what works for your body and gradually intensify the stretch.

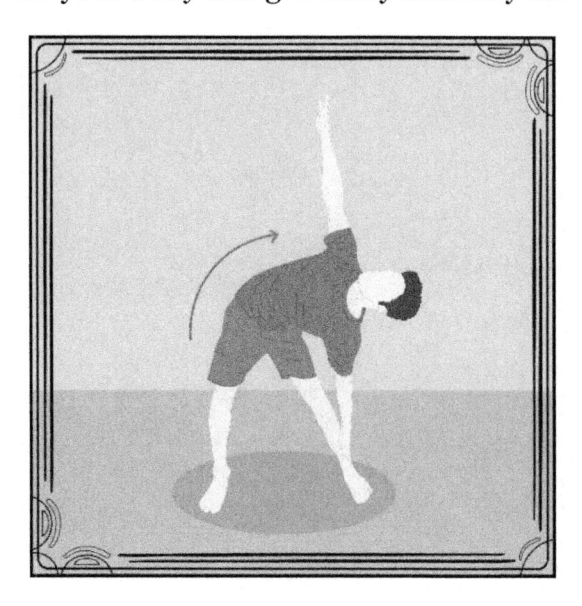

Instructions:

1. Stand tall and face forward. Step your legs in a wide stance of about four feet apart.
2. Turn your left toes out to the side and keep your right foot facing forward.
3. Open your arms out to your sides and shift your hips slightly to the right, bending at the waist.
4. Slide your left fingers down to your left ankle, and extend your right arm up toward the ceiling.
5. Look up toward your right hand and hold for 20 to 30 seconds.
6. Repeat on the opposite side. Perform three sets.

Seated Spinal Twist

Affected Areas:

- Abdomen: abdominal obliques, transverse abdominus
- Hips: adductors
- Buttocks: piriformis, gluteals

Good For:

A gentle turn of your spine in one direction, with support from your hands, is an easy way to give yourself a relaxing and passive stretch along your lower back, hips, and torso. This one is good for all ages and body types.

Level Up:

To challenge your balance, sit on a large fitness ball with your feet flat on the floor and about hip-width apart. As you move into your twist, press down through your feet into the floor and pull your core upward and inward.

Remember:

With cross-legged stretches, it's always good to alternate the upper and lower legs. This gives you an even balance throughout the body and a chance to work the nondominant body parts.

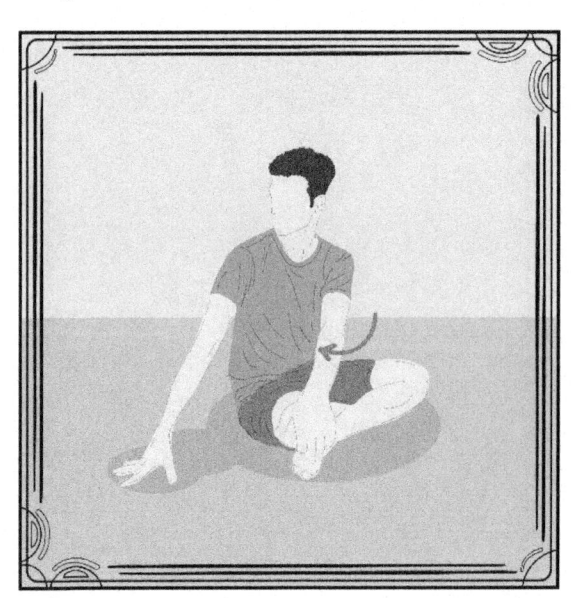

Instructions:

1. Take a seat on the floor or in a sturdy chair and loosely cross your legs.
2. Keeping your back upright, begin twisting your body to the right.
3. Reach your left arm across your chest to touch your right knee, and reach your right arm behind your right hip.
4. Turn your head to look over your right shoulder and hold for 30 seconds.
5. Repeat three times to each side.

Side Lunge

Affected Areas:

- Thighs: quadriceps, hamstrings, adductors
- Buttocks: gluteals, piriformis

Good For:

By shifting your weight to one hip and holding this lunge, you are activating the larger muscle groups that support your pelvis and hips while strengthening the smaller muscle groups. This isometric stretch may help mitigate lower-back pain and hip stiffness stemming from muscle weakness.

Level Up:

To advance this move, add a little weight. Hold a small weighted ball or dumbbell with both hands and raise it in front of your chest as you lunge to the side.

Remember:

It is important to maintain good form in this move. To protect your knee joint from overstretching, be sure that your bent knee does not extend farther to the side than your ankle. If necessary, step your feet wider apart to achieve this alignment.

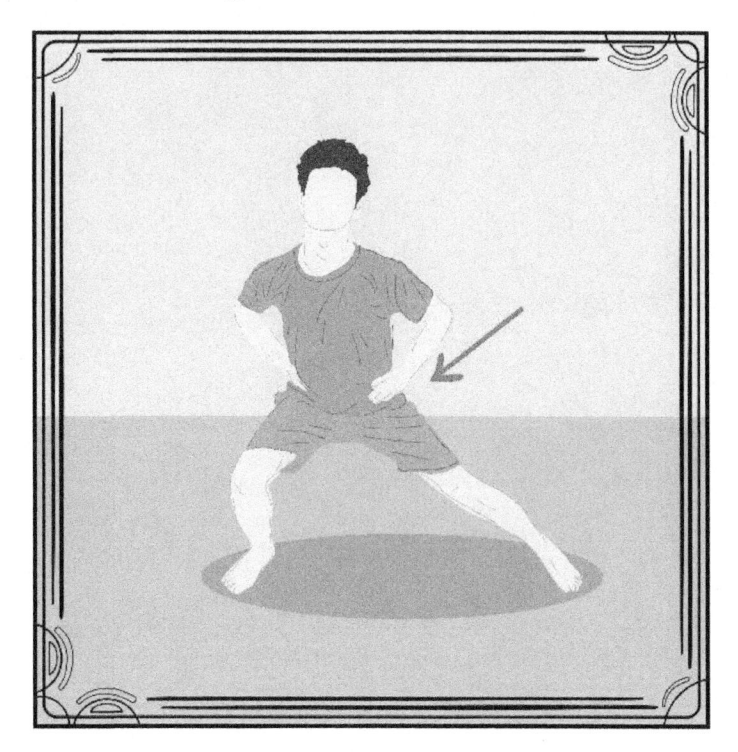

Instructions:

1. Begin by standing up straight. Step your legs open as wide as you can, and turn both feet slightly outward.

2. Place your hands on your hips and pull in your core muscles.

3. Slowly bend your right knee, keeping your back straight.

4. Take several deep breaths, holding the stretch for up to 30 seconds.

5. Repeat on the opposite side and perform three sets.

Legs, Knees, Feet & Ankles

Your legs are the foundation of your body, supplying support and stability. Toned, flexible muscles in your thighs, knees, calves, ankles, and feet can minimize aches and pains, improve posture, help prevent injuries, and speed recovery time after engaging in sports or workouts.

Toe Touch Standing

Affected Areas:

- Thighs: hamstrings
- Calves: gastrocnemius, soleus
- Buttocks: glutes

Good For:

Moving through this Toe Touch stretch is a great way to feel the connection of muscles from your hips, along the backs of your legs, and down to your feet. The inversion also helps get your blood flowing.

Level Up:

Hold a weighted ball in your hands to begin. As you bend forward, lower the ball toward your toes, allowing gravity to deepen the stretch along the backs of your legs.

Remember:

This stretch is great for anytime you feel tightness in the back of your legs. Find a comfortable location that allows you enough space to reach for your toes, and go for it.

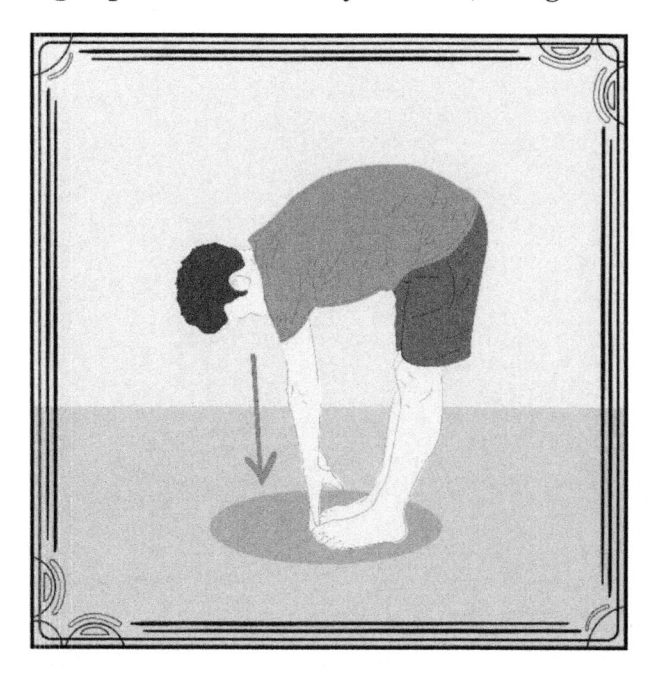

Instructions:

1. Stand up straight, lengthening your spine, and place your feet shoulder-width apart.
2. Lower your head and slowly curl your torso forward, one vertebra at a time, bending from your hips. Allow your arms to dangle loosely beneath you.
3. If you can, touch your toes, and breathe deeply, inhaling and exhaling.
4. Hold for 10 seconds.
5. Roll up slowly through your lower back and spine, and return to neutral position.
6. Repeat three to five times.

Standing Quadricep Stretch

Affected Areas:

- Thighs: quadriceps
- Shins: tibialis

Good For:

If you've ever been sitting for so long that when you stand up, the front of your hips feel stuck and cramped, this stretch may be beneficial for you. Release tension and stiffness from sedentary postures with this standing quadricep stretch.

Level Up:

For a stretch along your outer thigh and iliotibial band, grab your raised foot with the opposite hand. Allow your raised leg to turn out slightly, and bring your heel across to the opposite hip.

Remember:

Press your pelvis forward, and keep your hips flat to the front without arching your lower spine. If needed, use a wall or a chair for balance.

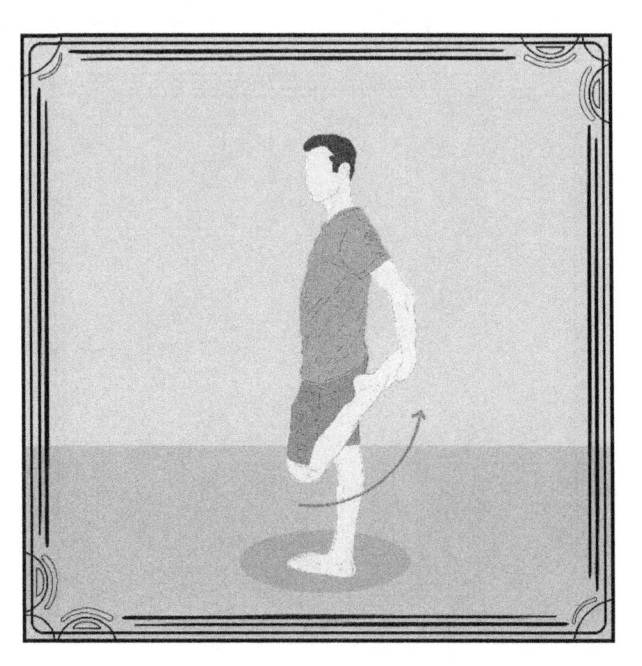

Instructions:

1. Stand straight with your feet together and engage your abs.
2. Bend your left knee, bringing your left foot up behind you.
3. Reach your left arm behind you, and wrap your hand around the top of your left foot. Bring your right hand onto your right hip to help with balance or let it hang at your side.
4. Pull your left heel in toward your left hip and hold for 10 to 15 seconds
5. Return to neutral position, and repeat two to three times on each leg.

Foot Sickle

Affected Areas:

- Shins: tibialis anterior
- Feet: extensors
- Toes

Good For:

Many of us spend hours on our feet daily and don't give them enough attention. Pain in your hips, knees, and lower back is sometimes related to how you stand on your feet. Try this isolated Foot Sickle stretch to rejuvenate your outer shins and ankles.

Level Up:

To get a deeper stretch through your ankle joint, hold your foot just below your toes. Pull the middle of your foot up toward you while keeping the support of the other hand on your shin.

Remember:

This stretch can be done either seated in a chair or with support of the floor. Take it wherever you go. Just remember to take off your shoes first so you can isolate the stretch accordingly.

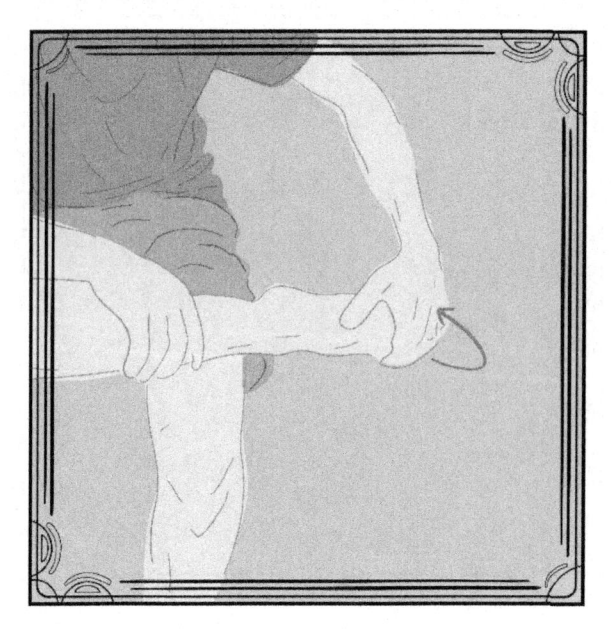

Instructions:

1. Find a comfortable seated position, and bring your right foot up to cross over your left knee.
2. Support your right shin with your right hand while you wrap your left hand around your right toes.
3. Isolating your toes and foot, pull your right toes toward your left shoulder.
4. Hold for 10 to 15 seconds and repeat on the opposite foot.
5. Perform three sets.

Toe Stretch

Affected Areas:

- Feet: extensors
- Arches of feet: plantar fascia
- Toes

Good For:

Your range of motion may vary significantly from toe to toe as you try out these easy Toe Stretch isolations. In addition to targeting your toes, this stretch series soothes tired ankles and arches. It's perfect for general foot pain and for cooling down overworked feet.

Level Up:

When stretching your toes, try moving them in a new direction. Instead of tugging them apart, push them up and down, working each neighboring toe against the other.

Remember:

Even though your toes are small, they play an important part in carrying and dispersing the weight of your body. Remember to care for them and be gentle when stretching.

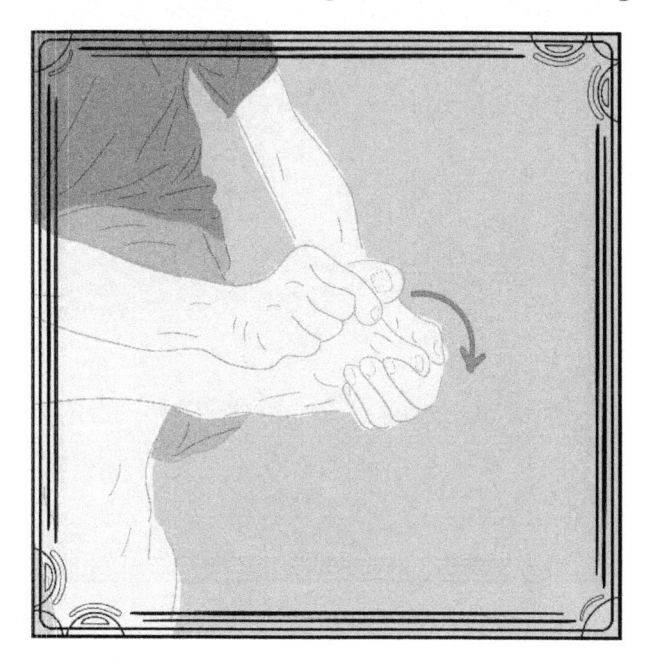

Instructions:

1. Find a comfortable seated position, and cross your right ankle over your left knee.
2. Begin by pulling your big toe away from your second toe.
3. Next, tug apart your second toe and middle toes.
4. Continue separating your toes this way down to your pinky toe.
5. Breathe deeply as you stretch, and repeat three to five times on each foot.

<u>High Knee Walking</u>

Affected Areas:

- Thighs: quadriceps, hamstrings
- Buttocks: gluteals

Good For:

This high knee stretch has many benefits. Not only are you stretching through your knees and upper legs, you're also improving strength, coordination, and circulation in your core, exterior leg muscles, and hip joints. This dynamic stretch is ideal for warming up before a run.

Level Up:

For an added challenge, strap on some light ankle weights and proceed slowly. This will serve to strengthen your quadriceps as well as improve your balance. Perform five repetitions on each leg.

Remember:

This is a simple exercise that you can do anywhere. It is especially useful as a warm-up before various sports and aerobic workouts. Engage your core to help you keep the movement fluid and controlled.

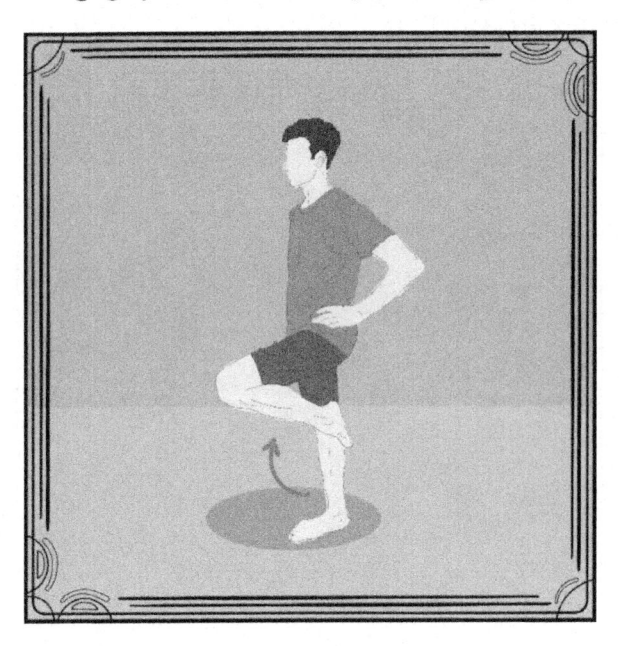

Instructions:

1. To start, stand upright with your feet positioned at a hip-width distance from each other. Place your hands on your hips.
2. Shift your weight onto your left foot, engage your core, and bring your left knee up high so that your hamstrings are parallel to the floor.
3. Lower your foot to the floor, stepping forward, and repeat with the opposite leg.
4. Continue walking for 10 repetitions on each leg.
5. Turn around and repeat three times.

Ankle Circles

Affected Areas:

- Shins: tibialis anterior
- Arches of feet: plantar fascia
- Toes

Good For:

When you move your body parts in a circular manner, you help promote circulation, mobility, and relaxation. Here, by isolating your ankle joint and moving it in a smooth circular motion through its maximum range, you can relax your tired, achy feet and enhance their flexibility.

Level Up:

Increase the range of motion by using your hand to assist your ankle through a wider circle. Place your left leg on your right thigh, and press your right palm against the sole of your left foot. Hold the sides of your arch and gently rotate your ankle in each direction.

Remember:

This stretch can be done just about anywhere, with or without your shoes on. If your feet are feeling achy or swollen, find a wall to help with your balance and circle your ankles a few times in each direction.

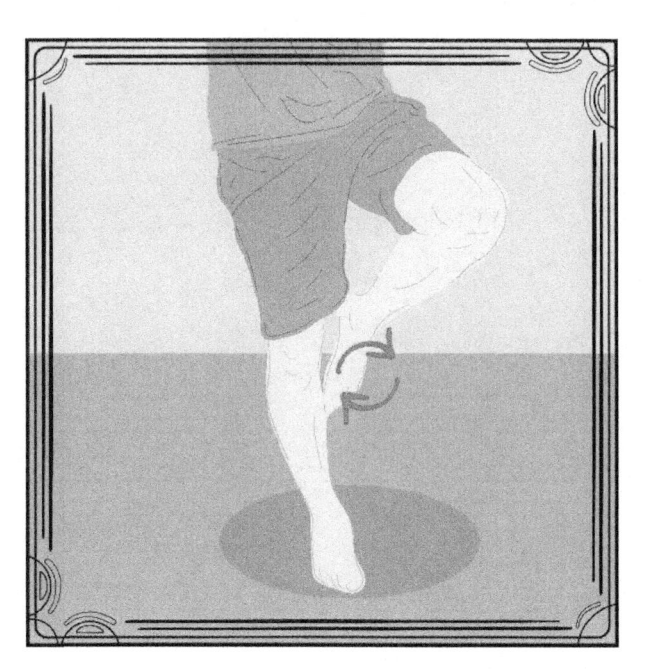

Instructions:

1. Assume a straight standing position, ensuring your feet are hip-width apart, and rest your hands on your hips.
2. Gently bend your right knee and raise your right foot off the floor.

3. Trace a small circle counterclockwise with your right foot by pointing your toes down to the floor, out to your right, up to the ceiling, and in toward your left leg.
4. Perform five circles, then reverse the direction, tracing a circle clockwise.
5. Repeat five times on each foot.

Wall-Assisted Calf Stretch

Affected Areas:

- Calves (gastrocnemius, soleus)
- Shins (tibialis anterior)
- Thighs (hamstrings)

Good For:

This intense stretch for your calves and Achilles tendons is a very familiar stretch that's especially popular with runners. With the support of a wall, you can push deeper into your lower leg while maintaining your balance the entire time.

Level Up:

Once you've found your comfort zone in the basic calf stretch, intensify the movement by turning your feet. As you stretch your right calf, shift your toes slightly outward to the right, then to the left. You'll feel the stretch along the sides of your calf.

Remember:

This is a stretch that should be done gently, with little force. Take care not to overstretch your calf muscles or Achilles tendon: Press your heel down slowly each time.

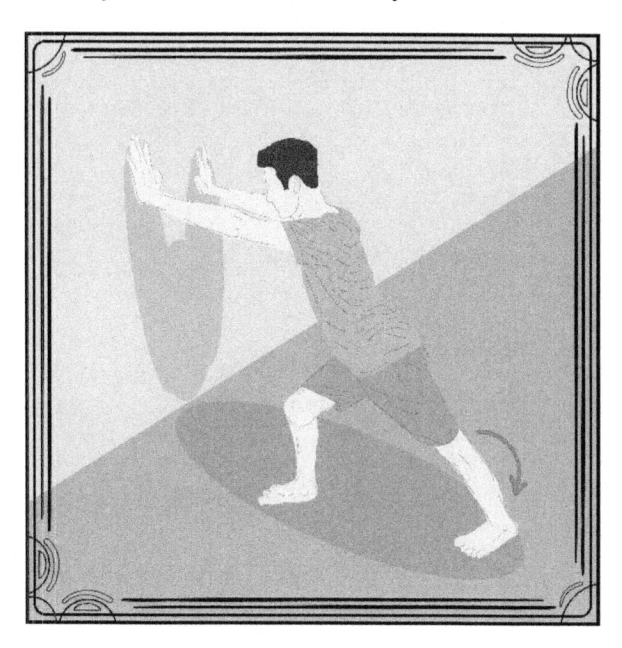

Instructions:

1. Stand straight facing a wall or another solid surface.
2. Place your hands on the wall at shoulder height to support your weight.
3. Bend your left knee, and step your right foot back about two to three feet behind you.

4. Straighten your right knee, and press your right heel down as you gently bend your left knee deeper.
5. Hold here for 20 to 30 seconds, return to neutral position, and repeat on the opposite leg.
6. Perform three repetitions.

Forward Lunge

Affected Areas:

- Thighs: hamstrings, quadriceps, adductors
- Buttocks: gluteals
- Shins: tibialis anterior

Good For:

The Forward Lunge reaches deep into your hips and opens the muscles around the front and the back of your legs and pelvis. Because you need to bend deeply through your hips, be sure to thoroughly warm up your back, hips, and legs before you attempt this exercise.

Level Up:

Intensify the stretch by holding the lowered position for 10 to 15 seconds.

Remember:

Protect your knee joints by making sure that you do not overextend your front knee. As you lunge forward, your knee should extend no farther forward than your ankle.

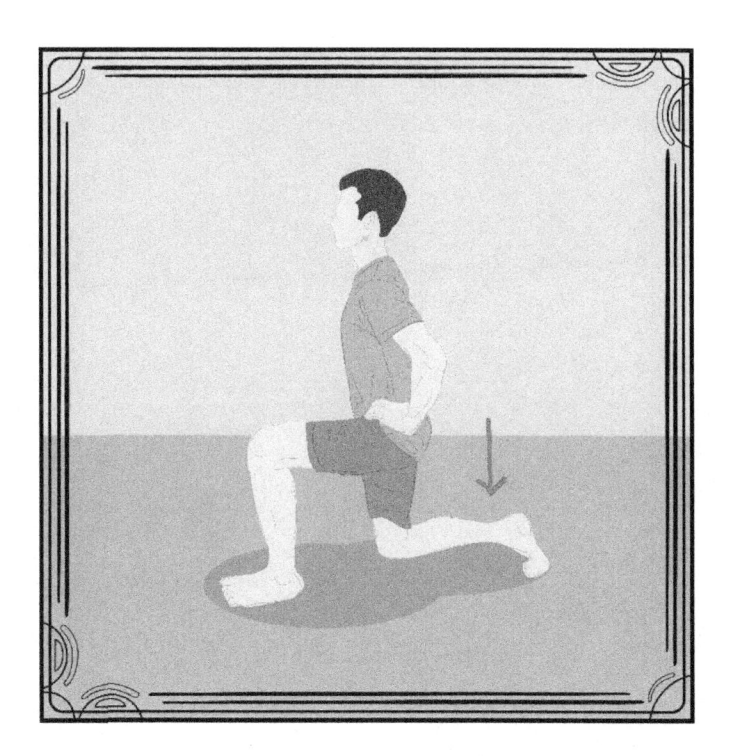

Instructions:

1. Start by standing tall, with your feet positioned hip-width apart, and place your hands on your hips.

2. Take a substantial step forward with your right foot, ensuring that you land with the heel making initial contact with the ground.

3. Transfer your body weight onto your right leg as you gently lower your right knee towards the floor.

4. Press your right heel into the floor to push you back to the neutral position.

5. Repeat on the opposite leg, and perform five times per side.

Chapter 4:
Building Balance and Stability

Balance training consists of exercises that help you develop and maintain your balance. Proprioception—the ability to detect the location, direction, position, and movement of the body and its many parts—can also be improved through balancing training. Balance training can be done inside or outdoors, in a gym or at home, and can be learned from a professional instructor or a website. Although balance training can benefit people of all ages, it is especially good for the elderly.

The Advantages of Balance Training

1. Reversing Age-Related Balance Loss

Our ability to balance deteriorates as we age. The amount of time a person can stand on one leg, for example, is an important predictor of lifespan.

Balancing is a difficult skill that requires the coordination of the brain, muscles, and components of the inner ear. The coordination between these three systems might degrade with time if you don't train and maintain balance, making it more difficult to stay upright and maintain appropriate posture.

Practice, on the other hand, keeps everything functioning as if your body were much younger, allowing you to avoid some of the balance concerns that come with aging. Dance is a fantastic technique to improve your balance.

2. Fall Prevention

Balance drills help you get better control of your core and limbs. Not only does this help you move more gracefully, but it also helps you avoid falling. When you have good balance, you can react more quickly to changes in body position, such as unanticipated height changes or rocks underfoot that you didn't notice.

Avoiding falls not only protects you from bodily harm such as broken hips, but it also enhances your self-esteem. You won't have to be concerned about falling every time you leave the house if you have decent balance. Even if you're young, having this unspoken awareness might help you feel more at ease in your surroundings.

You may react more rapidly to slips when your balancing system is working properly, making it less likely that you will fall.

3. Improving Your Posture

The ordinary individual has horrible posture as a result of poor movement form, a narrow variety of movement patterns, and an increasingly sedentary lifestyle. Hunched shoulders, anterior pelvic tilt, and restricted upper-back mobility are common restrictions. Part of the problem is that we don't undertake the essential balancing exercises to counterbalance the negative impacts of our way of life as a population.

Improving one's balance is beneficial to one's posture. It teaches you how to move in both static and dynamic positions, which are both natural to your human form. Outstanding balance necessitates excellent posture: the two go hand in hand.

4. Allowing For A Quicker Recovery Time After An Injury

Many persons who engage in athletic training sustain injuries, particularly to the legs and ankles. Much of what we know about balance comes from studies of persons who have suffered from lower-leg injuries. The findings of that study are fascinating: the more balancing drills people do, the faster they recover from injuries. Balance drills may even help to prevent injuries from occurring in the first place.

5. Better Coordination

Humans, like other animals in their natural settings, should have good coordination. However, modern civilization eliminates many of the physical labor that we might otherwise be required to perform. We rarely have to exercise balance because of our sedentary lifestyle. Our widespread lack of coordination is one of the consequences of this evolution.

Balance exercises, particularly dynamic balance drills like balance walking on rails, help to relegate balance to a reflexive reaction category. Finally, if you have good balance, you should be able to adapt naturally to almost any scenario without having to think about it.

6. Strengthening Your Muscles

Balance can help you develop your muscles and increase their power output swiftly. The greater the force they can exert, the faster you can sprint and the higher you can jump. Balance is beneficial in almost any sport that needs quick, acute, and powerful movements, such as boxing, as well as in the development of overall functional strength.

Balance Exercises
Side Leg Raise

Areas Targeted: Hips, abdomen, back, buttocks, outer thigh muscles, coordination, visual input, and proprioception.

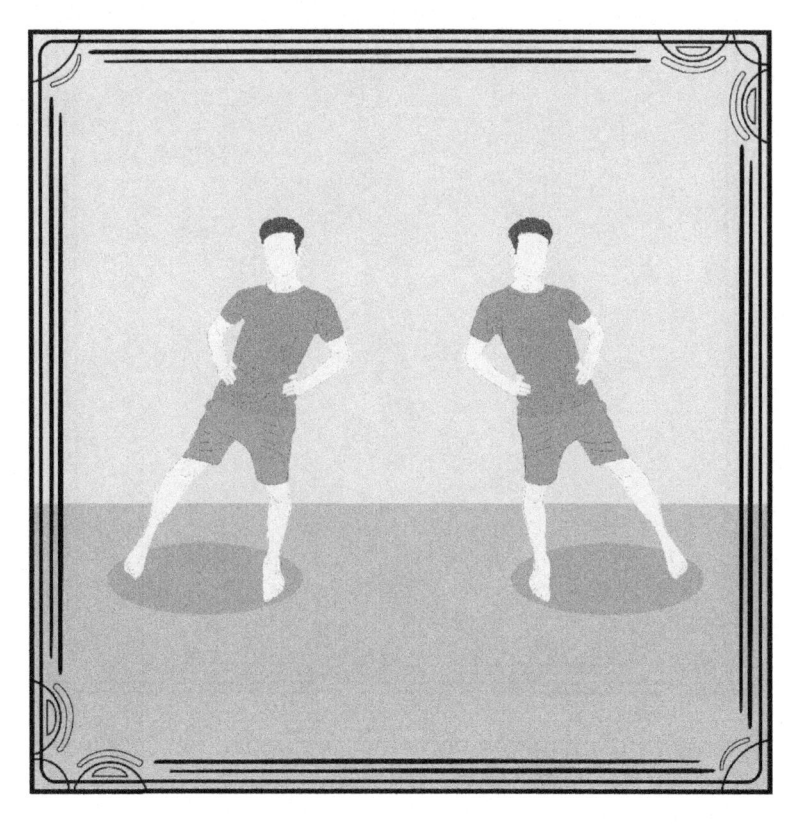

1. Stand with your feet hip width apart.

2. Place your hands on your waist with a bend at your elbows.

3. Lift your right leg out to the side keeping your knee straight.

4. Then lower your right leg back to the floor.

5. Lift your left leg out to the side keeping your knee straight.

6. Then lower your left leg back to the floor.

7. Continue alternating sides until you have completed eight raises with each leg.

Your torso will naturally lean a little to the opposite side of the leg that you are raising. However, be sure not to allow yourself to bend sideways at the waist. Also, avoid allowing your torso to lean so far that you feel you will topple over. If you are finding this difficult, you can perform this exercise standing in front of a kitchen counter, which you can hold for support.

Forward Heel Taps

Areas Targeted: Hips, ankles, knees, back muscles, coordination, visual input, and proprioception.

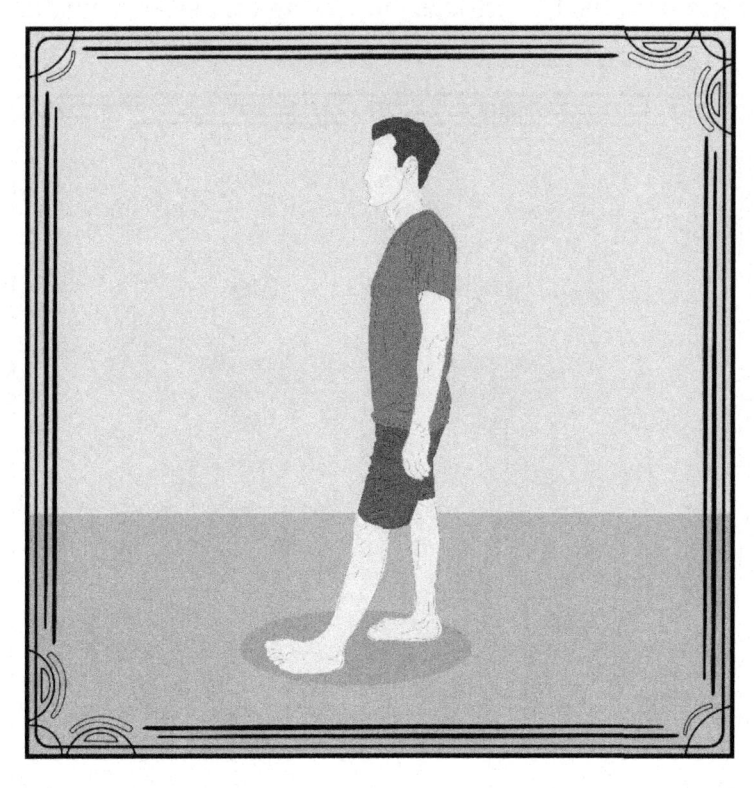

1. Assume a standing position, ensuring your feet are spaced at hip-width apart, and allow your arms to rest comfortably by your sides.

2. Step forwards with your right foot allowing only the heel to make contact with the floor.

3. Return your right foot to your original hip width stance.

4. Then step forward with your left foot allowing only the heel to make contact with the floor.

5. Return your left foot to your original hip width stance.

6. Continue alternating feet until you have completed eight heel taps on each side.

Aim to keep your ankle bent so that your toes point slightly upwards when you tap your heel on the floor. However, the more that you bend your ankle upwards, the more difficult this exercise will become. If you are finding this difficult, you can moderate the exercise by taking smaller steps or, if need be, by touching your heel to the opposite toes only and then returning to your hip width stance. And you can also perform this exercise standing next to a wall facing sideways onto it so that when you step forward you do so parallel to the wall and can support yourself by placing your hand against the wall.

Side Toe Taps

Areas Targeted: Hips, knees, ankles, abdomen, back, buttock muscles, coordination, visual input, and proprioception.

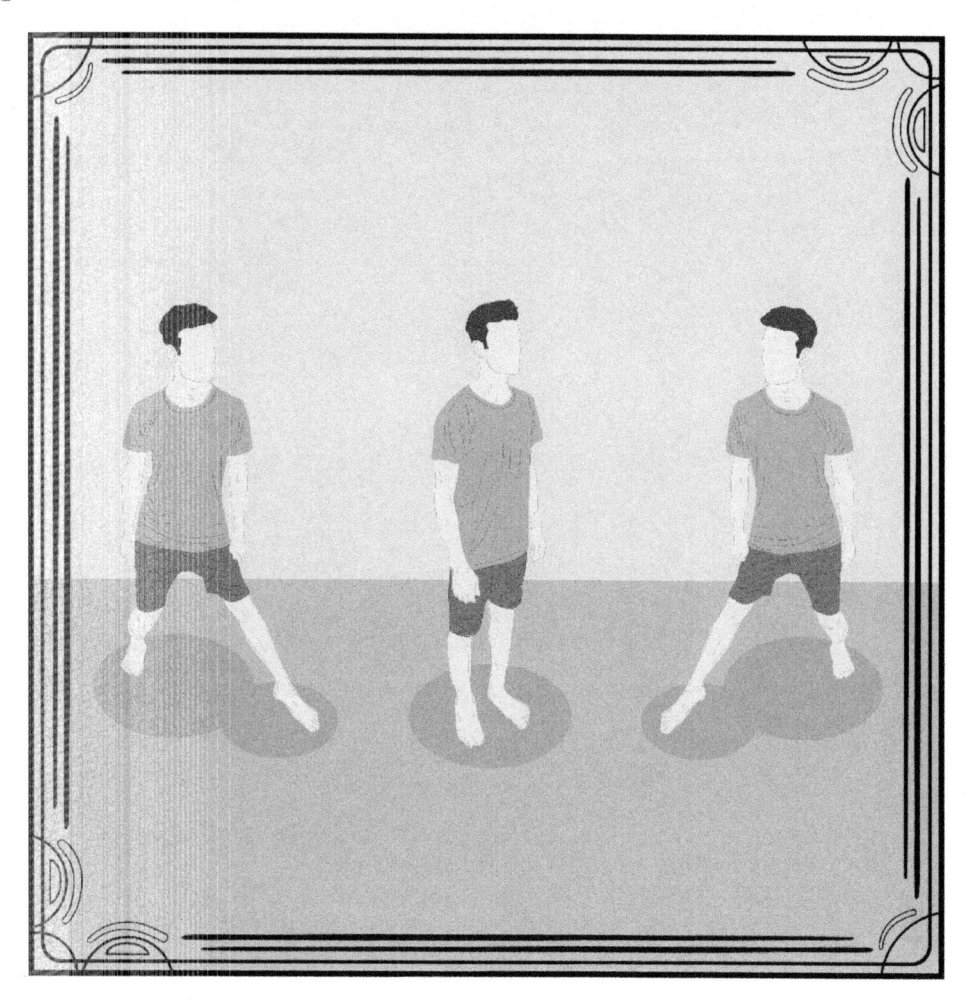

1. Stand with your feet hip width apart and your hands at your sides.

2. Step out to the side using your right foot.

3. Allow your left knee to bend so that your right step can be larger, tap your right toes to the floor at your side.

4. Bring your right foot back into your hip width stance.

5. Then step out to the side using your left foot allowing your right knee to bend so the step can be larger.

6. Bring your left foot back into your hip width stance.

7. Continue alternating sides until you have completed eight toe taps on each side.

Remember that the larger you make your steps, the lower you will need to dip by bending your opposite knee and the more difficult this exercise will become. In the beginning, if you are finding this exercise too difficult, you can stand in front of a kitchen counter and hold onto it for support. While doing this exercise, remember to keep your back straight and do not allow yourself to bend over towards either side.

Heel Raise

Areas Targeted: Ankles, knees, buttocks, calf muscles, and proprioception.

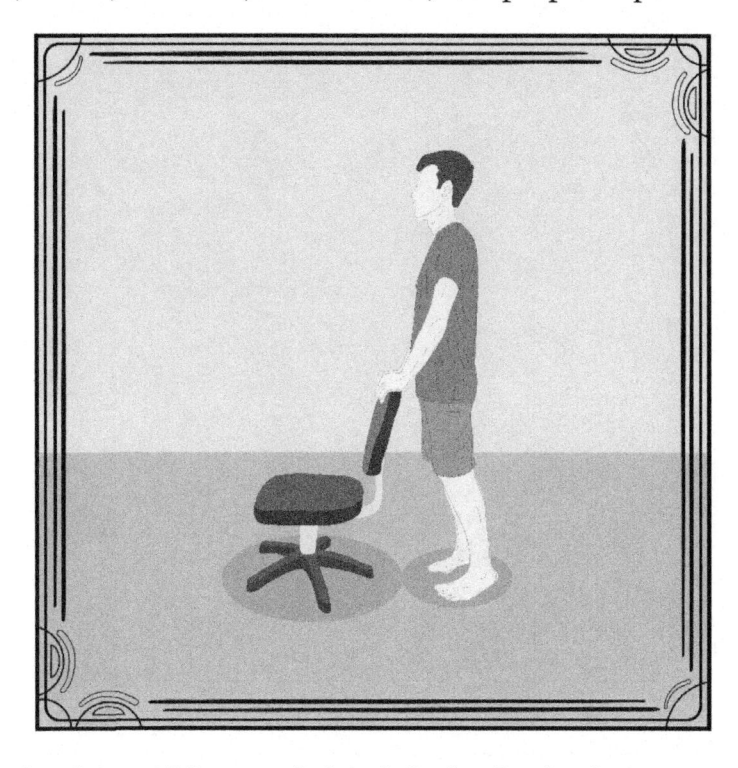

1. Stand with your feet hip width apart behind the back of a chair.

2. Hold the back of your chair with both hands for support.

3. Raise both heels off the floor at the same time until you are on your tiptoes.

4. Then lower your heels back to the ground.

5. Repeat this process 10 times.

If you are finding this exercise difficult, you can reduce the height that you raise your heel from the ground. For safety reasons, I recommend a chair be used for this exercise. Aim to keep your ankles, knees, and hips in a straight line up from the floor. By this, I mean avoid allowing your joints to bow out to the sides or into the middle whilst you raise your heels.

Toe Raise

Areas Targeted: Ankles, knees, buttocks, calf muscles, and proprioception.

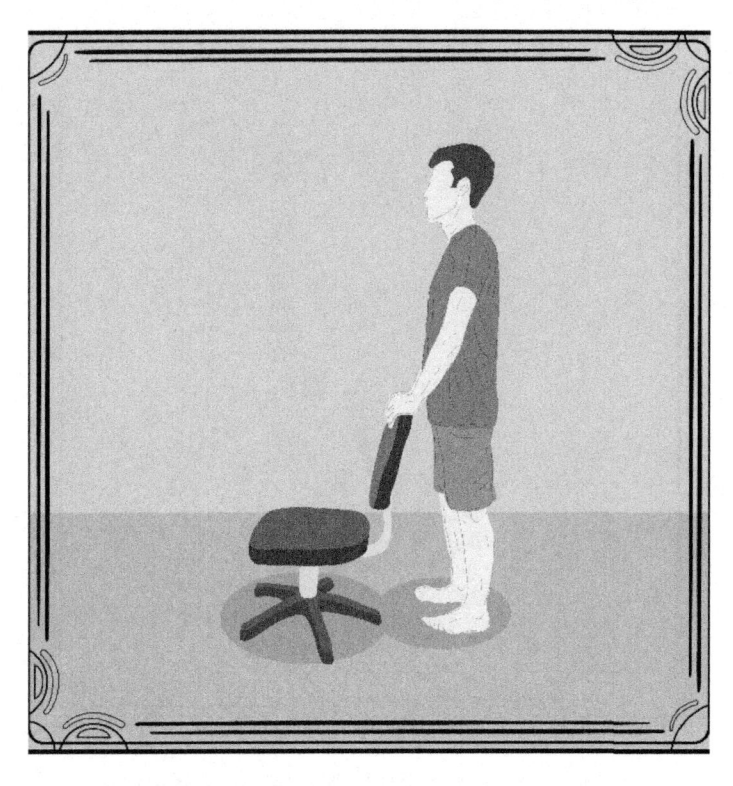

1. Stand with your feet hip width apart behind the back of a chair.

2. Hold the back of the chair with both hands for support.

3. Raise the balls of your feet on both sides at the same time so that you are lifting your toes towards the ceiling.

4. Lower your toes back to the floor.

5. Repeat this process 10 times.

You may find that you bend slightly at the hip to allow yourself to continue holding the back of the chair. A small bend is fine, but avoid a tendency to squat downwards. If you are finding this exercise difficult, remember that the higher you lift the toes, the harder it will become. Therefore, you can reduce the intensity when you first begin by doing smaller sized toe raises.

Lean Forward

Areas Targeted: Hips, abdomen, back, and shoulder muscles; coordination; visual input; and proprioception—particularly the balance structures in the ear.

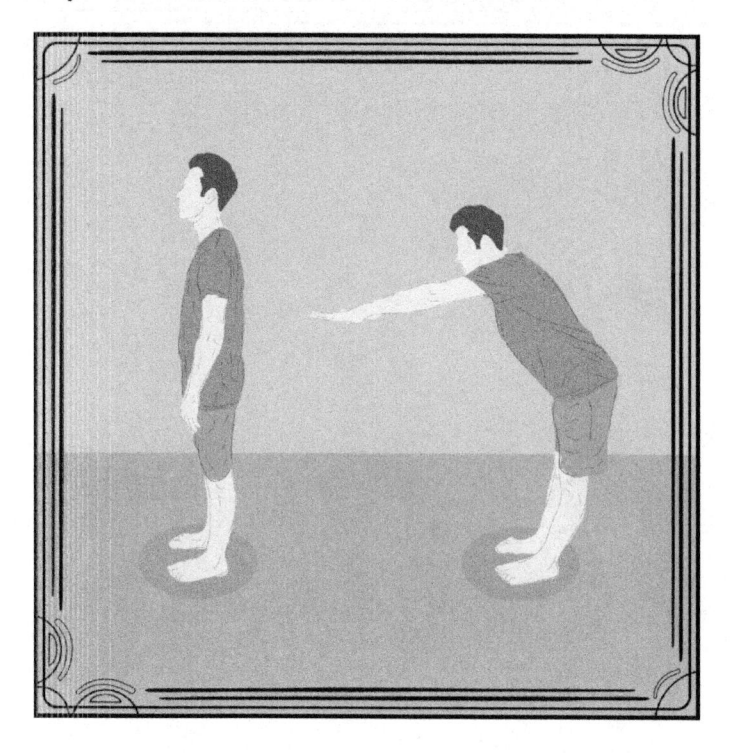

1. Stand with your feet hip-width apart.

2. Touch the inside edges of your wrists together with your fingers pointing forwards and raise your arms out in front of you until they are level with your shoulders.

3. Lean your torso forward until your shoulders cross an imaginary line made by the front of your toes.

4. Stand back upright and pause.

5. Then lean forwards again and repeat the lean eight times.

The further forwards that you lean the more off center your weight will be balanced and the more difficult the exercise will become. Remember that your hips might bend slightly backwards while you do this. A small bend is fine, but avoid allowing your hips to take over the motion. You want to reach forward and not squat backwards. If you are finding this exercise too difficult, you can adapt it by completing the leans without your arms stretched in front of you.

Seated Arm Lifts

Areas Targeted: Shoulder, upper arm, back, abdomen muscles, and proprioception.

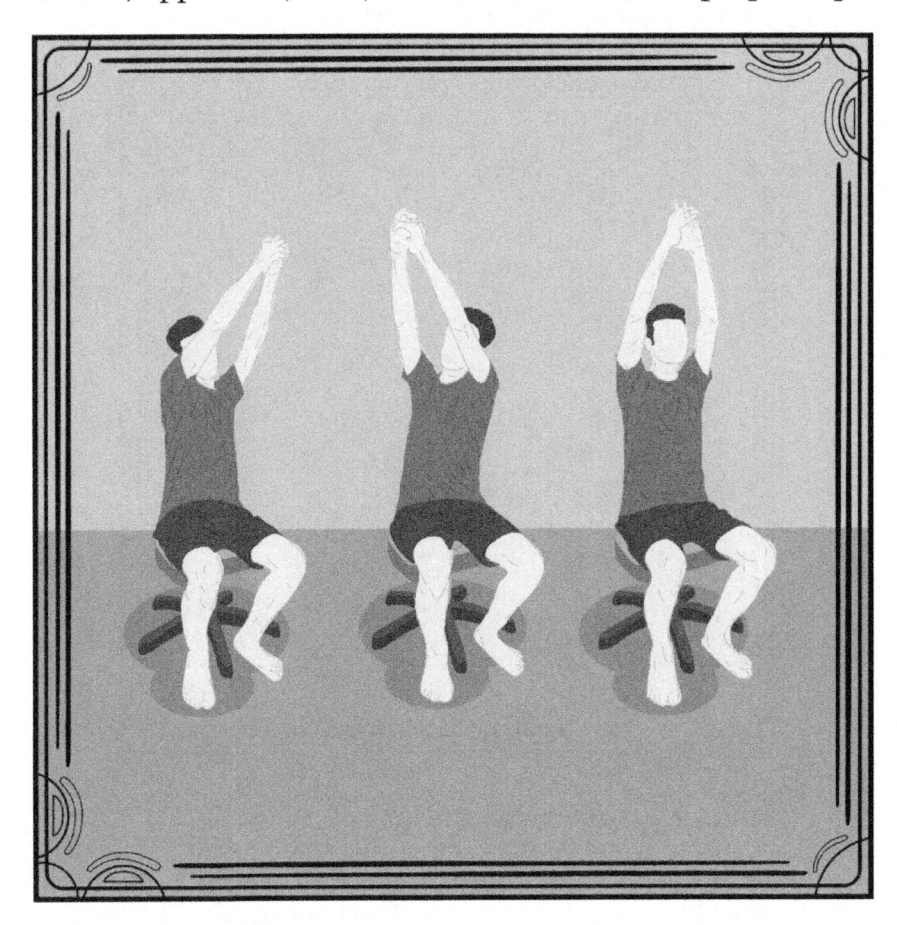

1. Sit upright in a chair with your feet hip-width apart.

2. Spread your knees slightly to allow your hands to touch the flat section of the seat in front of you.

3. Cup your right hand with your left hand and, with both hands together slowly raise your arms in front of you and then up over your head.

4. Slowly lower your arms.

5. Then raise them again. This time, keep them pointing forward but move slightly out to the side. Ending with your hands in the air above your head approximately in line with your right shoulder so that your back is curved slightly to the right.

6. Slowly lower your arms and then repeat, aiming to end with your arms above your head approximately in line with your left shoulder and your back slightly curved to the left.

7. Repeat this set of three times for a total of eight.

If you are struggling when you first start, you can make this exercise easier by only raising your arms halfway. If necessary, you can aim to only reach the height of your shoulders. Try to avoid twisting your torso. The aim is to keep your shoulders facing forwards as you lift your arms.

Seated Arm and Leg Lifts

Areas Targeted: Hips, thighs, abdomen, back, shoulder muscles, coordination, and proprioception.

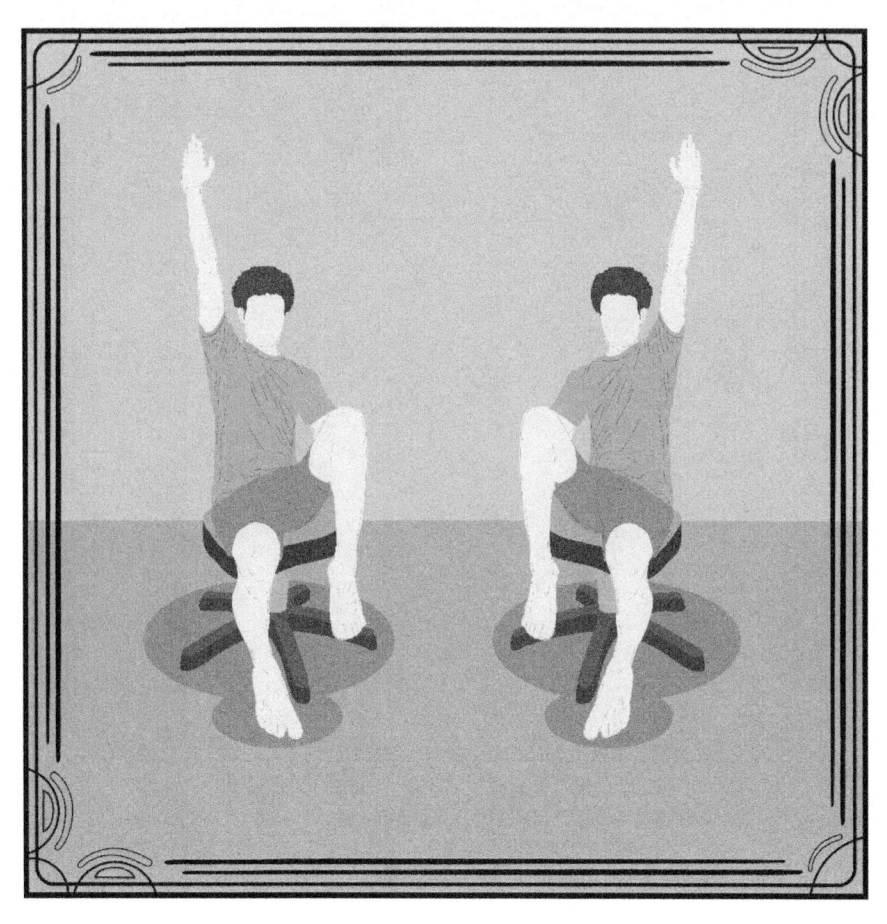

1. Sit in your chair with your feet hip width apart.

2. Raise your right arm and right leg at the same time, keep your arm straight and your leg bent at the knee at 90 degrees.

3. Lower your right arm and right leg at the same time, then swap sides.

4. Raise your left arm and left leg at the same time, keep your arm straight and your leg bent at the knee at 90 degrees.

5. Lower your left arm and left leg.

6. Continue alternating each side of your body until you have completed eight lifts on each side.

If you find it too difficult to alternate from side to side, you can make this exercise a little easier by completing eight repetitions on one side first and then switching to do eight repetitions on the other. Aim to lift your arm right up above your head and bring your knee as close to your chest as you can manage. Avoid allowing your torso to bend to the side or allowing your body to tip over to the side that you are currently raising in the air.

Torso Rotation Leg Openers

Areas Targeted: Hips, abdomen, back, thigh, buttocks muscles, and proprioception.

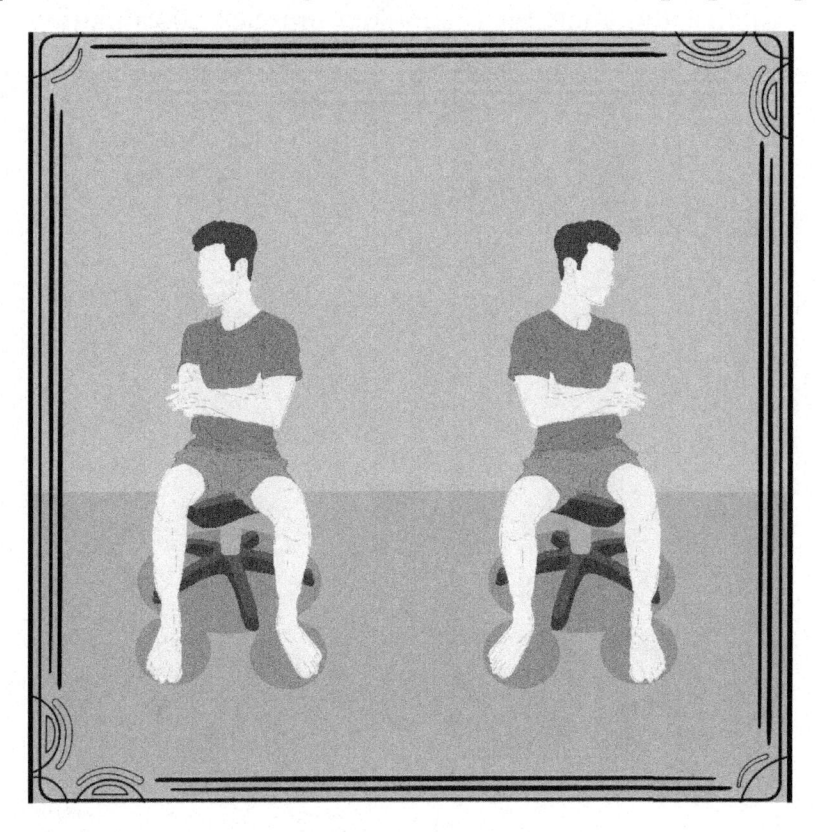

1. Sit upright in your chair with your feet hip apart.

2. Slide your left leg out to the side of the chair until your legs are at right angles to one another at the hip.

3. Then twist your torso to the right so that you are feeling a light stretch around your left hip area.

4. Twist your torso back to the center then return your left leg to its resting position in front of you.

5. Slide your right leg out to the side of the chair until your legs are at right angles to one another at the hip.

6. Then twist your torso to the left so that you are feeling a light stretch around the right hip area.

7. Twist your torso back to the center and then return your right leg to its resting position in front of you.

8. Continue alternating from side to side until you have completed eight twists in either direction.

Aim to twist your torso so that you can look over the back of the chair. It is fine if you cannot twist this far when you are first starting out. If you are finding this exercise difficult, you can support your upper torso by placing your arms on your extended knee and the back of the chair for support. However, avoid using your arms to pull your body into a twist. The movement should come from your hips and spine only. You may experience pain in your inner hip, especially if you stand or sit still for long periods of time. If this is the case, you can reduce the intensity by either reducing the degree of your torso rotation or by sliding your leg a shorter distance, thus reducing the angle between your legs.

Forward Reach to the Ankle Tap

Areas Targeted: Hips, abdomen, back, shoulders, buttocks, thighs, and calf muscles; coordination; visual input; and proprioception—particularly the balance structures in the ear.

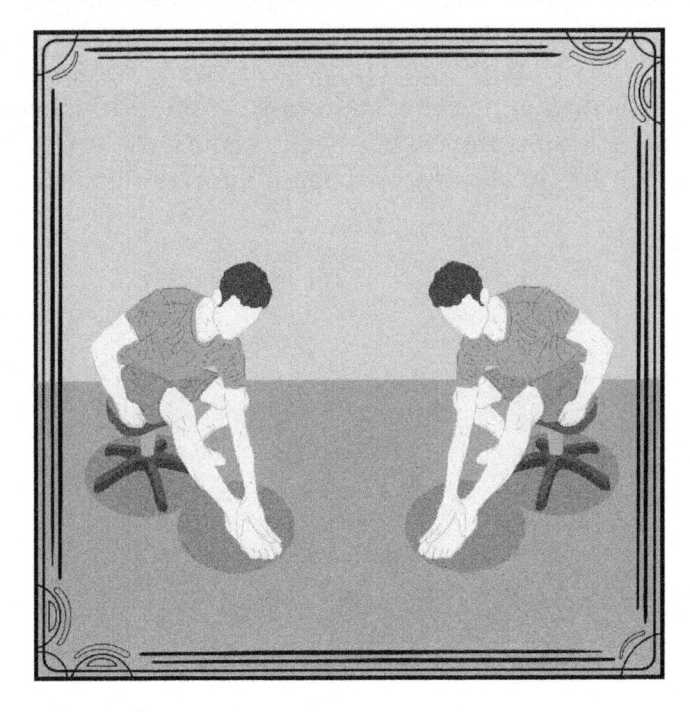

1. Sit upright in your chair with your feet hip width apart.

2. Gently slide your right foot forward while straightening your leg, making sure to keep the sole of your foot flat on the floor.

3. With your left arm, reach forward and over your center to touch the inside of your right ankle.

4. Return to an upright position then slide your right foot back towards the chair.

5. Now, smoothly slide your left foot forward, straightening your leg and maintaining the sole of your foot flat on the floor.

6. With your right arm, reach forward and over your center to touch the inside of your left ankle.

7. Return to an upright position then slide your left foot back towards the chair.

8. Continue alternating from side to side until you have completed eight ankle taps on each side.

You may experience some pain at the back of your knee, in your calves, or hamstrings if you are used to standing still a lot. To reduce this, you can reduce the distance that you slide your feet away from the chair and keep your knees slightly bent. And when you lean forward, be sure that most of the movement is happening at your hips and try to avoid curling your spine over your knee.

Chapter 5:
Strengthening for a Resilient Body

Strength training includes the performance of any exercise that causes our muscles to contract and create a force to move a load or weight; either our body weight and/or a specific external load, such as a barbell, dumbbells, kettlebells, etc. Other terms given to this type of exercise are "resistance training" and "weight training. Generally, they mean the same thing.

Benefits of Strength Training

It's never too late to experience the benefits of strength training. Those over 60 can benefit from strength training in multiple ways, including:

- Increased muscle mass
- Improved bone mass (density & content) and bone strength; decreasing the risk of osteoporosis
- Increased Resting Metabolic Rate; increasing energy expenditure and improved weight management
- Reduces excess body fat
- Increased functional capacity (your ability to carry out activities of daily living related to work and home life)
- Lower risk of developing functional limitations
- Lower risk of all-cause mortality
- Improved coordination, stability and balance
- Improved blood pressure in those who are pre-hypertensive or stage 1 hypertensive
- Increased self-confidence and self-efficacy
- Helps prevent falls

A multitude of studies have shown that regular strength training can significantly reduce the symptoms of age-related conditions, including:

- Arthritis
- Diabetes
- Lower back pain
- Osteoporosis
- Obesity
- Hyperlipidemia
- Dementia
- Depression

Strength Exercises

Forward Lunge

Additional Muscles Worked: Glutes, Hamstrings

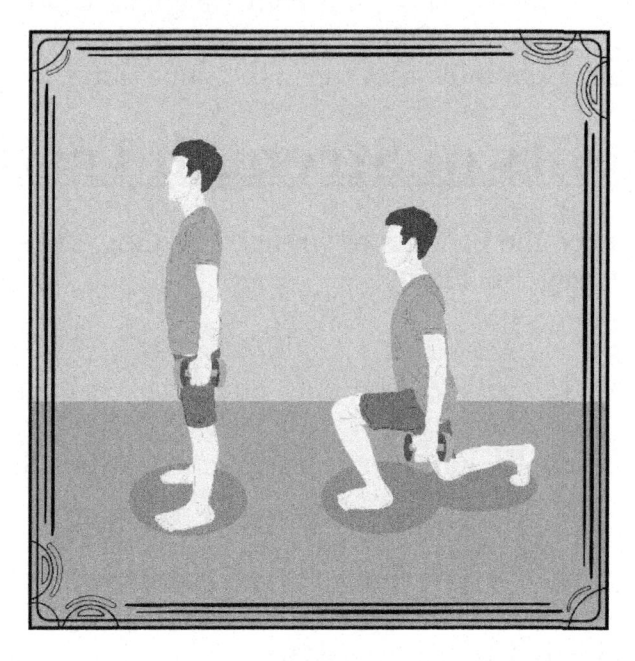

This exercise is a functional way to work your quads and calves because it is a similar movement pattern to walking. Lunges also help work your legs unilaterally (one leg at a time). Building strength unilaterally will help your bilateral exercises (squats and Deadlifts) become stronger.

1. Stand with your feet hip-width apart and toes facing forward. Hold dumbbells in both hands down by your sides with your back straight and shoulder blades squeezed together. If using a barbell, place it across your upper back along your shoulders.

2. Take a large step forward and bend both legs to 90-degree angles. Your back knee should hover just above the ground.

3. Drive out of your front heel to step back and return to the starting position. Repeat on the opposite side.

Lift Safely: Make sure your front knee stays behind your front toes as you lunge forward. Your front knee should track in the same line as your ankle and foot. Keep your back straight and chest high as you perform the movement.

Make It Easier: Do your lunges in place and without weight to learn the movement pattern. You can also put your hand against a wall or hold a stick for balance as you learn the movement.

Make It Harder: Perform walking lunges by stepping forward instead of returning to the starting position. To make it even harder, walk continuously without resetting in the middle of the movement by bringing your back leg straight through into another Forward Lunge.

<u>Lateral Lunge</u>

Additional Muscles Worked: Glutes, Hamstrings

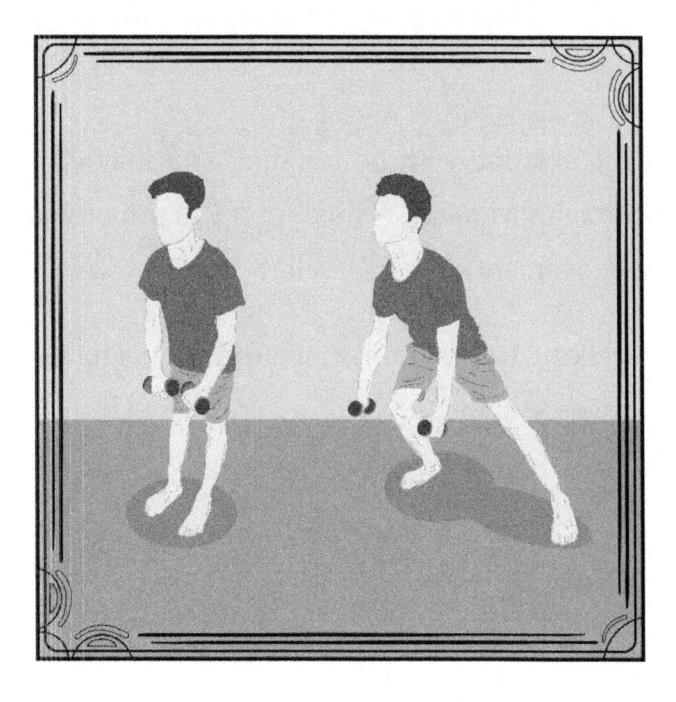

It is important to perform exercises in various planes of motion to mimic real-life movements. This exercise is similar to the Forward Lunge, but because it is in the frontal plane (moving side to side), it allows for different muscle activation. You will work more of your outer glute muscles and inner thighs.

1. Stand with your feet hip-width apart and your toes facing forward. Hold dumbbells at your sides in both hands with your back straight and shoulder blades squeezed together. If using a barbell, place it across your upper back along your shoulders.

2. Without turning your body, take a step out to your right and plant your right foot, toes facing forward. Bend your right knee to a 90-deg. angle as you lower your hips back and down like you're sitting in a chair. Keep your left leg straight and left toes pointed forward as you do this.

3. Push off the floor with the right foot, putting the weight in your mid foot, and return to the starting position.

4. Repeat on the left side.

Lift Safely: Keep your back flat and chest high as you perform this exercise. Keep your knee behind your toes and tracking over your ankle as you lunge. Your foot should be straight or slightly turned out when you step to the side, and your shoulders square. (Avoid bending your spine in the direction that you're lunging.) You want to keep your hips, knees, and ankles in alignment throughout the movement.

Make It Easier: Perform the exercise with no weights. You may also use a stick or wall to help balance yourself as you learn the movement. Adjusting the depth of your lunge so that you are not lunging as low will make the movement easier as well.

Make It Harder: Perform walking Lateral Lunges instead of staying in place. You can also increase the weight to progress this movement.

Bent-Over Row

Additional Muscles Worked: Biceps, Core

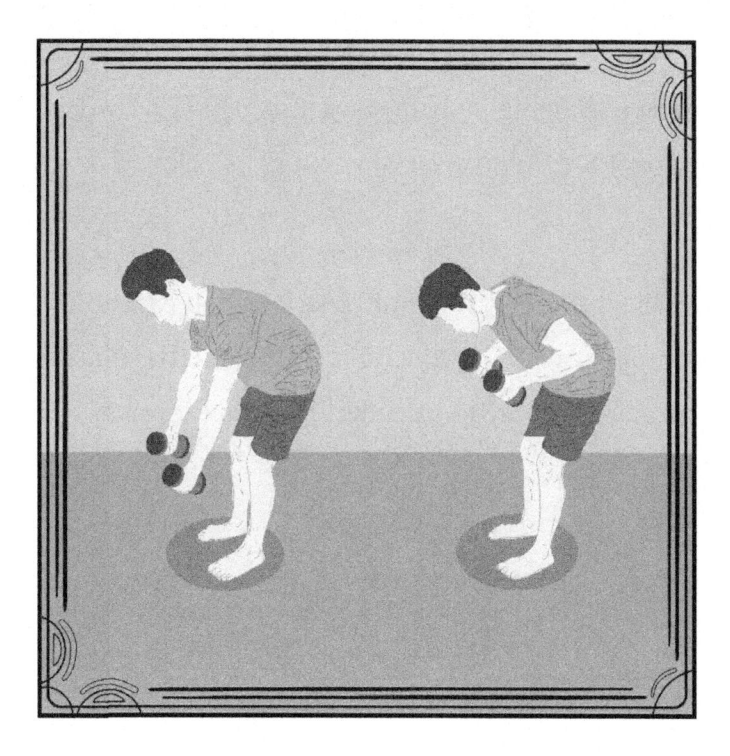

This movement specifically targets the rhomboids and assists in creating better posture. It's also a great exercise to help reinforce the deadlifting movement pattern. A strong Bent-Over Row will help improve the strength level of your other back exercises since you are engaging your middle and lower back muscles.

1. Stand tall with your feet under your hips, holding dumbbells at your sides or a barbell in front of you, hands gripping the bar just outside your thighs.

2. Hinge at the hips and lower your chest down toward the ground. You want to keep your back as straight and flat as possible as you do this. The weights should now be parallel to your chest with your palms facing each other.

3. Bend both elbows simultaneously and row the weights up until they reach your ribs. Squeeze your shoulder blades together at the top of this movement.

4. Slowly return the weights to the starting position by straightening your elbows.

5. Remain in the bent-over position until all repetitions are completed, then return to the starting upright position.

Lift Safely: Keep your back completely flat throughout the movement. Don't round the middle of your spine or arch your lower back while performing the movement. Engage the muscles in the middle of your back as opposed to using your upper traps. Do this by drawing your shoulder blades down and squeezing them together. Keep your shoulders as relaxed as possible and your neck in a neutral position.

Make It Easier: If it's too hard to hold the bent position, you can hold one dumbbell in one hand and use the other hand to support your weight on a chair. Use the chair to help stabilize your core and to find the correct neutral spine position needed for this exercise.

Reverse Fly

Additional Muscles Worked: Core, Shoulders

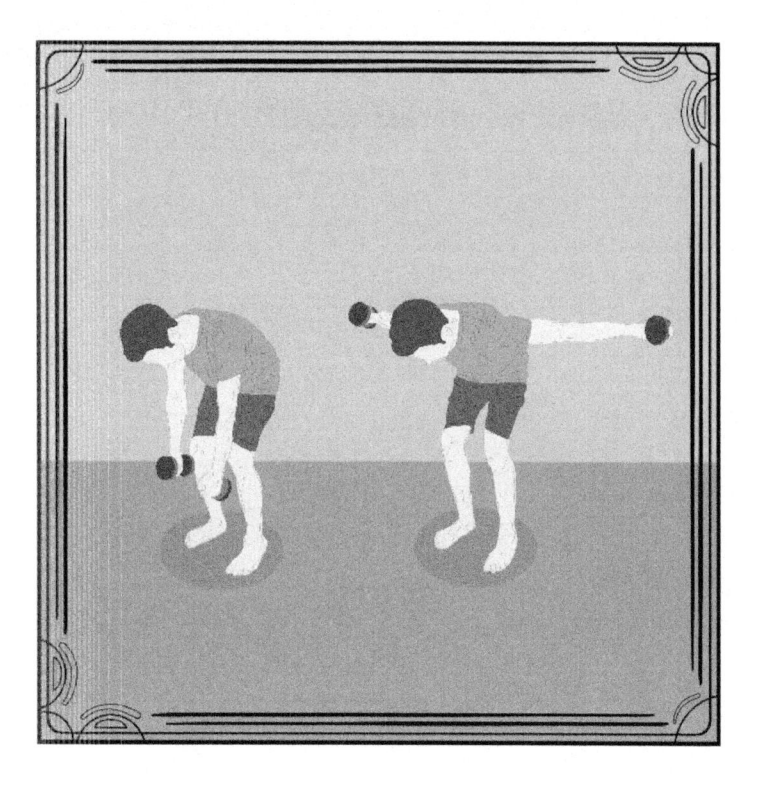

This exercise is really good for working some of the smaller muscles in and around your rotator cuff muscles. It's also a great way to improve your posture and overall strength. This movement is similar to Bent-Over Rows but is much more difficult due to the use of smaller muscle groups.

1. Position yourself by standing with your feet at a distance equivalent to hip-width, and grasp dumbbells on either side of your body.

2. Hinge at the hips and keep your back straight and flat as you lower your chest toward the floor. The weights should now be parallel to your chest with your palms facing each other.

3. While maintaining straight arms and slightly bent elbows, extend both of your arms out to the sides until they form a long, straight line. Picture yourself as a bird extending your wings to fly and squeeze your shoulder blades together at the top of the motion.

4. Return the weights to the center of your body just in front of your chest.

Lift Safely: Lift the weights in a slow, controlled motion. Avoid jerking your neck forward or raising your chest to try to use momentum to get the weights up. Don't overextend your arms. Perform the movement within a comfortable range of motion. Avoid arching your lower back.

Home Workout Hack: This is a great exercise to try with a resistance band. Simply hold the opposite ends of the band (as opposed to holding the handles). Pull the band apart like you're trying to rip it into two pieces.

Shoulder Press

Additional Muscles Worked: Biceps

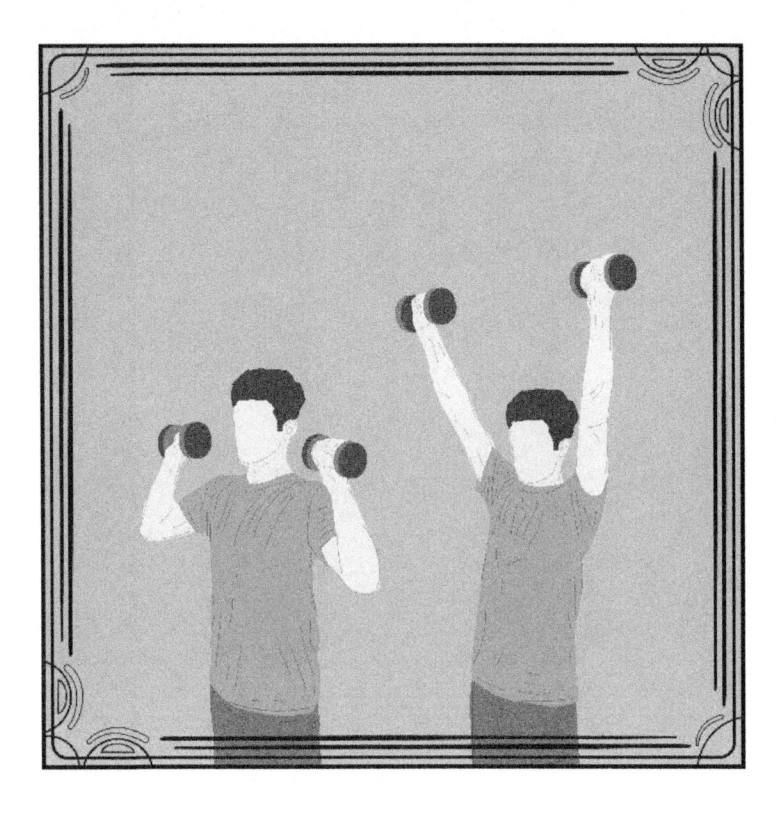

This movement is one of the fundamental movement patterns that humans develop from birth. It's one of the most common vertical press movements but should not be performed if you have a shoulder injury or have limited range of motion in your shoulders.

1. Stand with your feet shoulder-width apart holding dumbbells in your hands, or a barbell in both hands, and palms out.

2. Bring your elbows to shoulder height and align your wrists above your elbows, creating a 90-degree angle with your elbows.

3. Press the weights above your head and fully extend the elbows.

4. Return your arms to the starting position.

Lift Safely: Do not arch your lower back as you press the weights into the air. Keep your rib cage down and your neck neutral as you press the weights overhead.

Make It Easier: Press one dumbbell at a time into the air to require less core engagement.

Home Workout Hack: Perform this exercise using a resistance band. Simply stand on the band and press the handles over your head. Standing on the band with two feet will create more resistance than if you stand on the band with one foot.

Iron Cross

Additional Muscles Worked: Forearms

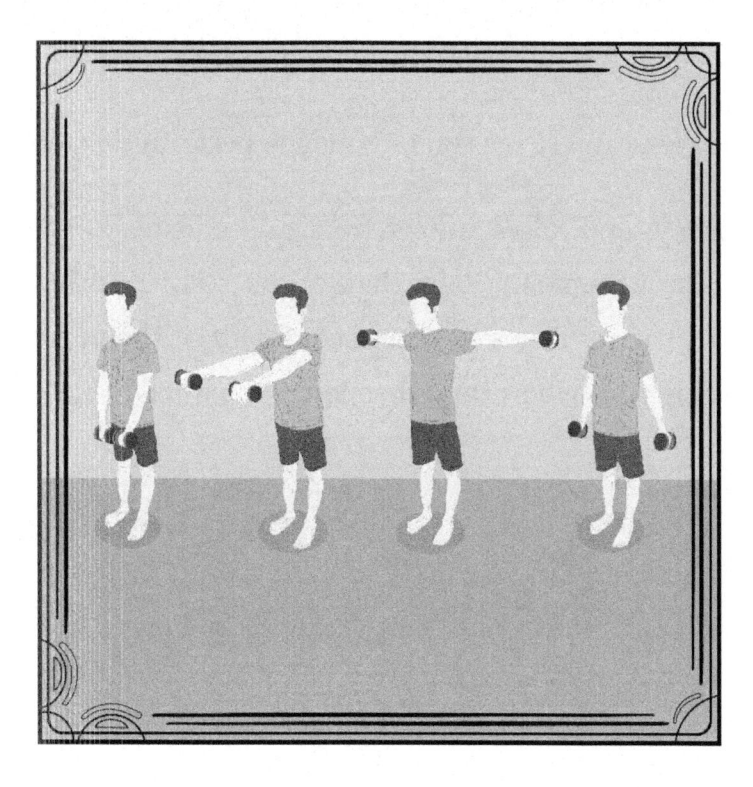

This exercise is very effective for working all three heads of your deltoid muscle, which is found in the top of your shoulder.

1. Stand with your feet shoulder-width apart holding the dumbbells in front of you and your palms down.

2. Raise your arms straight up in front of you to bring the dumbbells to shoulder height.

3. Keeping the dumbbells at shoulder height, extend your arms laterally (out to your sides) to form a T.

4. Lower both arms straight back down to the sides of your body.

5. Raise your arms straight up laterally, stopping when your hands are at the same height as your shoulders, to form that T.

6. Keeping the dumbbells at shoulder height, bring your arms together in the center of your body while keeping your arms straight.

7. Lower both arms back down along the front of your torso to bring the dumbbells back to the starting position.

Life Safely: Do not arch your lower back as you perform this movement. Do not raise your hands past the height of your shoulders at any point during this exercise.

Home Workout Hack: You can use resistance bands to perform this movement.

Make It Easier: Perform lateral raises and/or front raises instead of the full Iron Cross. Front raises are the first part of the movement. (Raise the weights to shoulder height and then lower them back down to your waist.) Lateral raises are the second half of the movement. (Raise your arms laterally with a slight bend in your elbows and then lower the weights back down by your sides.)

Upright Row

Additional Muscles Worked: Biceps

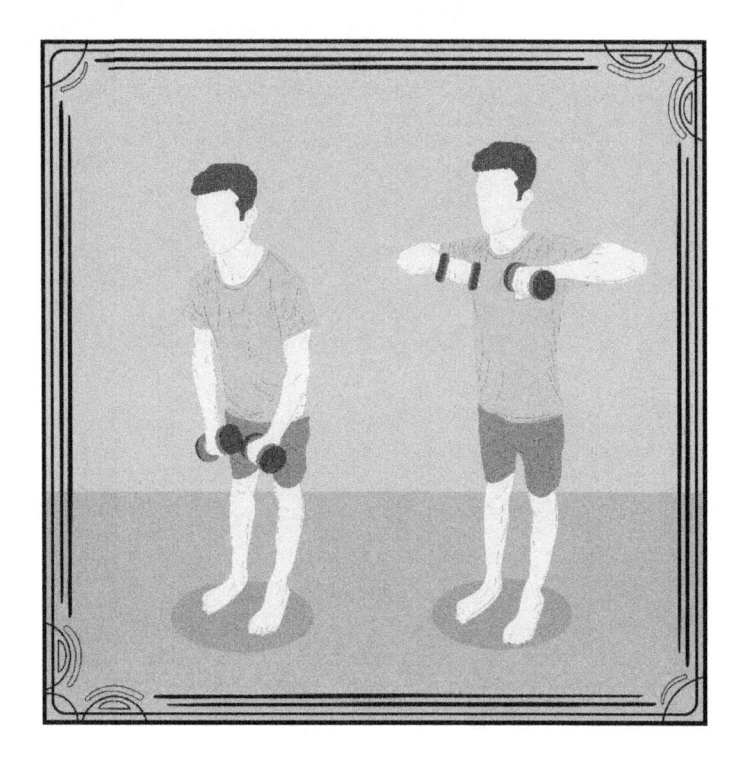

This exercise targets small muscle groups of the shoulder. It is a frontal plane movement that focuses more on the front and middle of your shoulders. This movement is popular among bodybuilders to help create more definition in the shoulders. It is not recommended if you don't have good posture or healthy shoulders.

1. Stand with your feet shoulder-width apart holding dumbbells, or a barbell, in front of your body at your thighs, hands shoulder-width apart, and with your palms turned toward your body.

2. Raise the weights up to the height of your chest by bending your elbows. Imagine yourself trying to create the shape of a clothes hanger with your elbows.

3. Return your arms to the starting position, keeping the weights close to your body throughout the movement.

Lift Safely: Do not arch your lower back as you perform this exercise. Stop if you feel any pinching or discomfort in the front of your shoulder. Think about squeezing your shoulder blades together on your back as you raise the weights up to chest height—similar to a wide row. This will help reduce some of the strain caused by the internal rotation of the shoulders.

Make It Easier: Lift one dumbbell at a time instead of simultaneously.

Home Workout Hack: You can do this exercise with a resistance band.

Chapter 6:
Customizing Your Routine

Developing a Personalized Stretching Routine

To design a personalized stretching routine tailored to your goals and preferences, follow these steps:

1. **Identify Your Goals:** First, define what you want to achieve with stretching. Are you aiming to improve flexibility, reduce muscle tension, or address specific issues like back pain? Knowing your objectives will guide the selection of stretches.

2. **Assess Your Current Flexibility:** Take a moment to gauge your current flexibility level. Try out a few basic stretches for major muscle groups, and note how far you can comfortably reach. This will serve as a starting point for tracking your progress.

3. **Consider Your Preferences:** Think about the types of stretches that resonate with you the most. Do you prefer gentle and slow stretches or more dynamic movements? Are you interested in yoga-based stretches, Pilates, or traditional static stretching? Tailor your routine to align with your interests to stay motivated.

4. **Factor in Time Constraints:** Recognize your daily time limitations. If you have more time available, a longer stretching session may be feasible, while a busy schedule might require a shorter, more efficient routine. Adapt the plan to fit your schedule.

5. **Begin with a Warm-Up:** Always start with a brief warm-up to prepare your body for stretching. Incorporate light cardio, like a brisk walk, or dynamic movements to increase blood flow and loosen up your muscles.

6. **Target Major Muscle Groups:** Your routine should include stretches that focus on major muscle groups, such as the hamstrings, quadriceps, calves, chest, shoulders, and back. Balancing upper and lower body stretches ensures overall flexibility.

7. **Address Specific Needs:** If you have specific areas of concern, add stretches that target those areas. For example, if you want to improve lower back flexibility, include stretches like the cat-cow stretch and seated forward bend.

8. **Balance Flexibility and Stability:** Combine stretches with stability exercises to enhance overall mobility. Consider incorporating core engagement or isometric holds during your routine.

9. **Adjust Intensity:** Modify the intensity of stretches based on your current flexibility level. Provide variations for each stretch to suit your comfort and ability.

10. **Focus on Proper Technique:** Ensure you use proper technique during stretches to prevent injuries and maximize benefits. Watch demonstrations to understand the correct form.

11. **Cool Down Effectively:** End your routine with a cool-down segment, featuring gentle stretches and deep breathing exercises. This will help relax your muscles and promote recovery.

12. **Progress Gradually:** Embrace a progressive approach, gradually increasing the duration or intensity of stretches as your flexibility improves. Celebrate your achievements along the way.

13. **Be Flexible with Your Routine:** Life can be unpredictable, so build flexibility within your routine. Modify it to fit your daily schedule while staying consistent with your stretching practice.

14. **Consistency is Key:** Emphasize regularity in your stretching routine. Even a few minutes of daily stretching can yield significant results over time.

Remember, this stretching routine is all about you and your unique needs. Regularly assess your progress and make adjustments as necessary to keep the routine enjoyable and effective. With a personalized approach, stretching will become a rewarding part of your daily life, promoting better flexibility, mobility, and overall well-being.

Sample Routine

Full-Body Routine (30 minutes total)

1. Neck Flexion - 1 minute
2. Wall-Assisted Upper-Back Stretch - 2 minutes
3. Arm Circles - 2 minutes
4. Wall-Assisted Bicep Stretch - 1 minute
5. Hip Twist - 2 minutes
6. Toe Touch Standing - 1 minute
7. Side Leg Raise - 1 minute
8. Forward Heel Taps - 1 minute
9. Forward Lunge - 2 minutes
10. Lateral Lunge - 2 minutes
11. Bent-Over Row - 2 minutes
12. Reverse Fly - 2 minutes
13. Shoulder Press - 2 minutes
14. Triangle Pose - 2 minutes
15. Seated Spinal Twist - 1 minute
16. Toe Stretch - 1 minute
17. Side Lunge - 1 minute
18. Prayer Hands - 1 minute
19. Seated Arm and Leg Lifts - 2 minute
20. Neck Extension - 1 minute

Upper Body Routine (10 minutes total)

1. Wall-Assisted Chest Opener - 1 minute
2. Arm Circles - 1 minute
3. Elbow Circles - 1 minute

4. Extended Palm Press - 1 minute
5. Posterior Arm Cradle - 1 minute
6. Shoulder Circles - 1 minute
7. Bent-Arm Fly - 1 minute
8. Tricep Stretch - 1 minute
9. Neck Flexion Assisted - 2 minute

Lower Body Routine (20 minutes total)

1. Toe Touch Standing - 2 minutes
2. Side Lunge - 2 minutes
3. Forward Lunge - 2 minutes
4. Lateral Lunge - 2 minutes
5. Hip Twist - 2 minutes
6. Triangle Pose - 2 minutes
7. Standing Quadricep Stretch - 2 minutes
8. Wall-Assisted Calf Stretch - 2 minutes
9. Ankle Circles - 1 minute
10. Toe Stretch - 1 minute
11. Foot Sickle - 1 minute
12. High Knee Walking - 1 minute

Tracking Progress

You need to assess your results at least six weeks after you start your exercise program and continue monitoring your progress every few months. Doing this will help you determine the effectiveness of your exercise program or if you require to make any changes.

To do this, you can design a simple activity log table showing the activities you cannot do on one side and progress on the other. Here is a sample you can use.

Daily and Mobility Activities	Progress After Six Weeks
I can walk to the mall without pain in my leg.	
I can climb stairs easily	
I can easily bend to pick something off the floor	
I can step over things without difficulty	
I can lift heavy objects without experiencing pains	
I no longer have weight issues.	

Stick the activity log next to your exercise schedule so you can easily revisit it after six weeks.

Rewarding Yourself

However long it takes to see the changes, even if it's just walking half a mile without pain in your legs or joints, every milestone is worth a reward.

You can reward yourself by going out with friends or buying the latest workout gear. Book yourself a massage if that keeps you going and looking forward to the next workout session!

Conclusion

In conclusion, this book has been an enlightening exploration of the transformative power of stretching exercises for individuals over 60. Throughout this book, we have delved into the myriad benefits that a consistent stretching routine can bring, not just to our physical bodies but to our spirits and overall well-being. As we come to the end of this journey together, let us take a moment to recap the main highlights and celebrate the profound impact that stretching can have on our lives.

The benefits of stretching exercises for seniors over 60 are truly remarkable. We have discovered that flexibility is not merely a physical attribute but a gateway to a life of greater vitality and independence. Through regular stretches, we have learned how to maintain joint health, improve balance, and reduce the risk of injuries, thereby allowing us to fully engage in the activities we love.

Moreover, stretching has shown us the path to mental clarity and emotional well-being. Embracing mindful movements, we have learned to let go of stress, anxieties, and worries, finding solace in the present moment. As we reconnect with our bodies and movements, we have unlocked the ability to approach life's challenges with grace and resilience.

Throughout this journey, we have emphasized the importance of perseverance, and listening to our bodies. Remember, this is not a race to reach a certain level of flexibility; it is a journey of self-discovery and self-compassion. Each step you take, no matter how small, is a triumph worth celebrating. As we tune into our bodies' needs and limitations, we develop a deeper understanding of ourselves, fostering a sense of empowerment that extends far beyond the realm of stretching.

Perseverance is the key to unlocking the full potential of this journey. Some days may be more challenging than others, and that's okay. What matters most is the commitment to yourself and your well-being. Embrace the setbacks and hurdles with the knowledge that they are part of the process. Stay consistent, and you will witness the gradual transformation that arises from the dedication to your stretching routine.

As we conclude this book, I extend my heartfelt gratitude to each and every one of you, dear readers, for embarking on this path of improved flexibility, vitality, and a joyful aging experience. Your dedication to self-improvement and your willingness to embrace new possibilities are truly inspiring.

Remember that you are not alone on this journey. We are a community of like-minded individuals, supporting and uplifting one another as we age gracefully. Cherish the connections you have made, both with yourself and with others, throughout this process. Let us continue to celebrate the joys of staying active, engaged, and connected in the later years of life.

May this book serve as a guide, a source of inspiration, and a reminder that the path to a fulfilling life is never-ending. As you continue your stretching journey, always remember to honor your body, nurture your spirit, and savor the moments that make life truly extraordinary.

Appendix
Additional Resources

Books:

- "Stretching for 50+" by Karl Knopf: This book offers a comprehensive guide to safe and effective stretching exercises specifically designed for older adults.
- "The Joy of Stretching" by Jessica Matthews: While not exclusively for seniors, this book provides a range of stretching exercises suitable for all ages and fitness levels, including modifications for seniors.

Websites:

- National Institute on Aging (NIA) - Go4Life: The NIA offers a comprehensive website with exercise tips for older adults, including stretching exercises. Visit https://go4life.nia.nih.gov/ for helpful resources.
- ElderGym: ElderGym offers a variety of stretching exercises and workout routines designed for seniors to improve flexibility, balance, and overall mobility. Website link: https://eldergym.com/
- Senior Fitness With Meredith: Meredith is a certified personal trainer who creates workout videos specifically for seniors. Her YouTube channel features various exercises, including stretching routines and low-impact workouts. Website link: https://www.seniorfitnesswithmeredith.com/

Videos:

- Gentle Stretching for Seniors, Beginner Exercisers: (https://www.youtube.com/watch?v=kfjVFQWWiZw)
- Improve Your Flexibility: 7 Effective Stretching Exercises for Seniors and Beginners (https://www.youtube.com/watch?v=yI4hnt0IXDw)
- Exercises for Seniors - Stretching Exercises for Seniors - Exercises for the Elderly (https://www.youtube.com/watch?v=YGRje8p5gbc)

Glossary of Terms

Balance: The ability to maintain equilibrium and stability during movements or while in a stationary position.

Cool-Down: Gentle exercises or stretches performed after a workout to gradually reduce heart rate and return the body to a resting state.

Flexibility: The range of motion around a joint or a group of joints. Flexibility exercises help improve the ability to move joints freely and effectively.

Gentle Stretch: A mild and controlled stretch, suitable for seniors and individuals with limited mobility.

Hamstrings: A group of three muscles located at the back of the thigh that play a crucial role in leg movement and bending the knee.

Hip Flexors: A group of muscles that enable hip flexion, which involves lifting the leg towards the torso.

Overstretching: Stretching beyond the natural range of motion, which can lead to injury. It is essential for seniors to avoid overstretching and listen to their bodies during stretching exercises.

Proprioception: The body's ability to sense the position, location, orientation, and movement of its limbs and muscles without relying on vision.

Range of Motion (ROM): The extent to which a joint can move in various directions.

Repetition (Rep): The completion of one full movement of an exercise.

Sets: A group of repetitions performed consecutively, with a rest period in between each set.

Warm-Up: Gentle movements or exercises done before stretching to increase blood flow and prepare the muscles for stretching.

Frequently Asked Questions

Here are some frequently asked questions about stretching exercises for seniors:

1. **Is it safe for seniors to start stretching exercises, especially if they haven't exercised regularly before?**

Yes, it's generally safe for seniors to start stretching exercises, even if they haven't exercised regularly before. However, it's essential to begin slowly and gently to avoid injury. Consult with a healthcare professional before starting any exercise program, especially if you have pre-existing health conditions.

2. **Can stretching exercises help improve flexibility and range of motion in seniors?**

Yes, stretching exercises can significantly improve flexibility and range of motion in seniors. Regular stretching helps to maintain or regain flexibility, which is essential for everyday activities and maintaining independence.

3. **What are some simple stretches that seniors can do at home?**

Seniors can do a variety of simple stretches at home, including neck stretches, shoulder rolls, seated hamstring stretches, calf stretches, and ankle circles. Gentle yoga poses and tai chi movements are also great options.

4. **How long should seniors hold a stretch?**

Seniors should hold a stretch for about 15-30 seconds. Avoid bouncing or overstretching, as this can lead to injury.

5. **Can stretching exercises help with arthritis pain and joint stiffness?**

Yes, stretching exercises can provide relief from arthritis pain and joint stiffness. Gentle stretches can improve blood circulation, reduce muscle tension, and ease joint discomfort.

6. **Should seniors stretch before or after exercise?**

It's generally recommended to perform a warm-up before exercise, which can include light cardio and dynamic stretches. After the workout, seniors can do static stretches as part of their cool-down routine.

7. **How many times a week should seniors do stretching exercises?**

Seniors should aim to do stretching exercises at least 2-3 times a week. Daily stretching is even better, as it can enhance flexibility and mobility.

8. **Can stretching exercises help prevent falls in seniors?**

Yes, regular stretching exercises that improve flexibility and balance can help reduce the risk of falls in seniors.

9. **What are the best stretches for seniors with back pain?**

Some effective stretches for seniors with back pain include the cat-cow stretch, seated spinal twist, and gentle lower back stretches.

10. **Are there any stretches to avoid as a senior?**

Seniors should avoid overly aggressive or intense stretches that may strain their muscles or joints. It's important to listen to their bodies and modify stretches as needed.

11. **Can seniors do partner stretches or should they stretch alone?**

Seniors can do partner stretches if they have a partner who can provide support and assistance. Otherwise, they can perform stretches alone using safe and effective techniques.

12. **What time of day is best for stretching?**

The best time for stretching is whenever it fits into your schedule. Some people prefer stretching in the morning to awaken their bodies, while others find it beneficial before bedtime to relax.

13. **What should I do if I feel pain during stretching?**

If you experience pain during stretching, stop immediately. Stretching should not cause sharp or intense pain. Mild discomfort is normal, but listen to your body and avoid pushing too far.

Scan the QrCode and downlowad the ebook '*Joint Health Mastery: A Comprehensive Guide to Nutritional Excellence*'. Your bonus is waiting for you!

Printed in Great Britain
by Amazon